DIETARY INTERVENTIONS IN AUTISM SPECTRUM DISORDERS

DIETARY INTERVENTIONS IN AUTISM SPECTRUM DISORDERS

Why They Work When They Do,
Why They Don't When They Don't

KENNETH J. AITKEN

Jessica Kingsley Publishers
London and Philadelphia

First published in 2009
by Jessica Kingsley Publishers
116 Pentonville Road
London N1 9JB, UK
and
400 Market Street, Suite 400
Philadelphia, PA 19106, USA

www.jkp.com

Library of Congress Cataloging in Publication Data
A CIP catalog record for this book is available from the Library of Congress

British Library Cataloguing in Publication Data
A CIP catalogue record for this book is available from the British Library

ISBN 978 1 84310 939 6

Printed and bound in the United States by
Thomson-Shore, 7300 Joy Road, Dexter, MI 48130

For my wife Ros,
and my daughters
Natasha and Chantal.

Many of the things we need can wait. The child cannot. Right now is the time his bones are being formed, his blood is being made and his senses are being developed. To him we cannot answer 'Tomorrow'. His name is 'Today'.

Gabriela Mistral

Contents

PART III THE SIMPLE RESTRICTION DIET (SRD)

RESOURCES

FIGURES AND TABLES

How to Use This Book

Unless you are prepared yourself to profit by your
chance, the opportunity will only make you ridiculous.
A great occasion is valuable to you in proportion as you
have educated yourself to make use of it.

Orison Swett Marden

Not everyone with an autism spectrum disorder (ASD) requires help
but many do. This applies as much to dietary interventions as it does to
other aspects of everyday life. This book sets out to explore why
looking at diet can be helpful to some and explores the issue of which
people it might help.

We begin by examining some general ideas about diet and about
dietary changes that have taken place in recent human history. This sets
the scene for considering the main dietary approaches that have been
advocated for, and by, many people with an ASD.

There is a brief summary of each approach that we discuss, an
explanation of what it purports to do, an examination of the extent of
the evidence for and against, and any reported problems resulting from
adopting the approach. Where it is available, information is given on
relevant publications, web resources and support groups.

The rest of the book deals with a general approach to dietary intervention drawing on a common principle that underpins the more
successful methods that have been advocated to date. Starting from
what we call the Simple Restriction Diet (SRD), we go on to describe
how to implement the approach, how to evaluate whether it seems to be
of benefit, and how to move, with appropriate advice and support,
from this quite limiting initial diet to identifying specific factors that
may be affecting you, your child, your loved one or your client, and how

to adopt a least restrictive beneficial diet which can be adopted for the longer term.

The dietary intervention discussed here may be all that is required to address biomedical issues or may not even be required at all. It may be that this approach provides a starting off point but that more detailed assessments and further interventions are required. As many component aspects of the general approach are readily available from websites, downloadable papers and readily accessible books, these are referenced as appropriate rather than adding unnecessary padding here.

PART I

DIETS, ASDS AND DIETARY INTERVENTIONS

CHAPTER 1

Introduction to Diet and ASDs

I take the view, and always have, that if you cannot say what you are going to say in twenty minutes you ought to go away and write a book about it.

Lord Brabazon of Tara (1884–1964)

First and foremost, this is a book about dietary factors in ASD, how they can affect mood and behaviour, how understanding the bases to different dietary approaches can help to identify whether a particular dietary intervention may be worth trying, and how, if you implement a diet, to tell whether it has done any good. It provides a mixture of theory, evidence and practical advice together with some forays into why some of the evidence base is not as strong as we would ideally like it to be.

This is not a book on how to help obese people with ASD to control their weight. Weight loss may result from some of the approaches we discuss but is not the primary focus. A wide range of diets is advocated for weight loss, and the evidence is often confusing and contradictory (a recent brief overview of 50 of the more popular dietary interventions for weight control can be found in Rodriguez 2007).

Neither is this a book on how to cope with behavioural issues in food avoidance (an introduction to this topic can be found in Ernsperger and Stegen-Hanson 2005). I see many ASD individuals who have problems with weight control, but almost as many are underweight as are overweight. Food refusal and difficulties with the introduction of new foods are common problems in ASD (see Cornish 1998), so in adopting any new dietary intervention, finding strategies to deal with these difficulties is important. Often, however, such difficulties are biological in origin and lessen as dietary management begins to show benefits – for example, zinc depletion is common and severe zinc depletion can markedly affect someone's sense of taste. As body zinc levels improve, a wider range of foods becomes palatable.

Dietary treatment interventions are often difficult to understand, complicated to implement and expensive to maintain. Despite these hurdles, and the limited clinical expertise and support typically made available, many families try hard to implement a variety of specialized diets and frequently claim that they see improvements as a result.

Dietary approaches to ASD are today being used by many and can have major beneficial effects. Most are largely safe and can correct a range of physiological differences. Diet should be corrected first before considering any detailed biomedical assessments or other complementary or alternative approaches. Investing in tests and supplements as a starting point may be both expensive and wasteful where a change of diet might have achieved the same or a similar effect. Differences in diet can result in findings suggesting a particular metabolic difference is present when it is not or could mask a real difference/ deficiency which is already being addressed.

I am not arguing that every person with an ASD has a dietary problem that requires to be addressed; many people do not. There is now a steadily growing literature written by people with ASDs who appear to fit well in society and use their differences to their own advantage (see, for example, Robison 2007, for an eloquent autobiographical account of a highly successful person with an Asperger syndrome diagnosis).

The evidence to date does, however, suggest that such problems are not uncommon. Here, we review and discuss the literature that suggests that such differences affect many individuals who have an ASD, and suggest a method for starting to address this issue.

The ancient Greek term *diaita* stood for 'way of life' or 'way of being' and had far broader connotations than the term diet as used today. We typically use diet as a term for a way of cutting down on food after periods of overindulgence in order to try and lose weight rather than as a lifestyle choice.

The Autism Research Institute (ARI), founded by Bernard Rimland, has for many years collected questionnaire data from families of people with autism on the treatments that have been tried and the families' perceptions of how useful they have been. From the ARI questionnaire data returned by families to the Institute in San Diego, dietary interventions are consistently reported as showing good results (see www.autism.com).

In their assessment of diet outcomes, the ARI asks families to rate whether the treatments they have tried have made the person worse, had no effect or resulted in an improvement. Their most recent survey data is shown in Table 1.1 with respect to effects of dietary interventions:

Table 1.1 Recent ARI diet outcomes

	Worse	No change	Better	Numbers reporting
Candida diet	1%	41%	58%	71
Sugar-free diet	3%	48%	49%	207
Feingold diet	0%	45%	55%	96
CF-GF diet	3%	27%	70%	237
Rotation diet	3%	37%	60%	65
SCD	3%	33%	64%	33

It has to be remembered that this is not a 'head-to-head' comparison of approaches. The different diets are often begun for very different reasons. Benefits found from one might not have been looked for from another that could have proven to have the same or a similar effect. In addition, they are being reported on by families who have enough motivation to complete a detailed record form and return it, so are a relatively highly motivated and self-selected group. Whether similar levels of success would be found for an unselected group of people with ASD, or if the recording forms had been completed by someone independent, is impossible to say. What can be said is that within this group the perception of those completing this information is of a high level of success from adopting dietary interventions. This compares to relatively low levels of reported success for more conventional psychopharmacological treatments.

There are many excellent and well-qualified dieticians and nutritionists who know about the normal metabolism of foods, their calorific values, vitamin and mineral content, and the effects of specific metabolic conditions such as phenylketonurea (PKU). Few however are knowledgeable about the dietary treatments that are advocated for ASDs, about whether they are backed by sensible theories, or about the evidence for their safety and efficacy. Interest among dieticians in ASD is steadily growing (Peregrin 2007).

I am not for a moment trying to minimize the importance of the other food-related issues mentioned above – dietary self-restriction can have severe consequences and can result in blindness (Uyanik *et al.* 2006), developmental delay (Casella *et al.* 2005) or worse. In the Uyanik *et al.* paper cited, the child they discuss developed progressive visual loss due primarily to lack of vitamin A (his serum level was 10 µg/l with a normal range of 360–1200 µg/l). This was as a direct result of keeping to a diet from the age of four to eight years that consisted of nothing except fried potatoes and water. A high proportion of ASD children will self-restrict and, as a consequence, they can become deficient in a range of essential nutrients (Cornish 1998).

The general literature on dietary approaches to weight loss and to a range of other conditions is vast. I have tried, where possible, to draw attention to some of the material from this general literature here, where it is relevant. In contrast, the literature on dietary approaches to ASD is relatively sparse. I hope that the coverage given here deals with the major approaches, which have been advocated to date in a reasonably fair and non-judgemental fashion, and access to the resources which will enable anyone to explore the issues farther.

I hope that, as a minimum, this book will provide an introduction to, and a clearer understanding of, various dietary approaches that are advocated for those with ASD. I hope it can also offer some reassurance that there is a literature on, and a rationale for, many of these approaches and there are clinicians who are both competent in the area of ASD and who believe that biobehavioural approaches such as these can be important. It should also be clear that many of the issues are complex, and that rigid adherence to some of these approaches can lead to difficulties which might not at first be obvious.

I also introduce and discuss methods that in the individual case should help to assess their effects. It is often as important to be able to demonstrate that something has worked as it is to have achieved the desired outcome.

> Please bear in mind the various factors raised later in the book that are important to check on before starting – like any other approaches which can have positive effects there is also the possibility of negative ones.
>
> A number of the issues covered here are fairly complex, and have been included to provide a basis for informed discussion with a supportive clinician rather than as definitive information.
>
> Topics such as possible effects of diabetes, phenylalanine metabolism, celiac disease, ketogenics and oxalates will fall in this category for many readers.
>
> A number of the possible difficulties arising from diets that are covered here are not dealt with systematically in other books which have dealt with dietary aspects to ASD, and it is as important to be aware of these as it is of the positive effects.

Why do we eat what we do?

In general, mankind, since the improvement of cookery,
eats twice as much as nature requires.

Benjamin Franklin (1706–1790)

Let's start by raising a theme to which we will return – the history of our present human eating patterns and how our nutrition has changed.

From the beginnings of recorded time, gathering, preparing and eating food have been shared social activities (Jones 2007). For all of us from birth, our nutrition, whether we are breast or bottle fed, is part of an interaction with at least one other person (see Trevarthen and Aitken 2001). Throughout the world, gathering food (whether by harpoon, spade, boomerang, or shopping trolley), food preparation, and food consumption are inherently social activities. The requisite skills are often learnt in groups or passed on from parent to child. Differences in social functioning cut to the heart of what makes those with autism special. Often difficulties with this shared process of nutrition are central to how those with ASD present from the earliest early stages of life.

How we eat and how we learn to eat are important, so is what we eat. As we will see, our diet has undergone huge changes over recent generations, in part as a result of globalization of food production and a consequent degree of homogenization of what is consumed.

Sugar

Sugar was not used in Europe until Crusaders brought it back from the Holy Land in the 11th century. Cane sugar was first used in India, where there is evidence of sugar cane cultivation as early as 10,000 BC. The process of crystallizing sugar from sugar cane, however, was not discovered until around 350 AD (Adas 2001).

Although honey has been used at least since 2100 BC when it is mentioned in contemporary Sumerian and Babylonian cuneiform texts, it was highly prized and recorded when given in tributes along with precious stones and metals. It is unlikely that honey would have been produced commercially in large enough volume to be used as a significant food source for the general population.

Sugar use made its way to Persia when the Emperor Darius conquered parts of Western India in 510 AD and discovered the 'reed which makes honey without bees'.

Sugar beet was a much later discovery, first being used to make sugar in 1747.

Sucrose consumption in England has risen steadily and inexorably, through lowering costs, and the steadily increasing volume of imports. From an average consumption of 6 kg per person per year in 1815 it had risen to the staggering level of over 50 kg per person per year by 1970 (Cleave 1974).

When you consider that the average Western person currently obtains some 550 calories per day from sugar alone (this would have been only 66 calories in 1815), it is not surprising that waistlines are steadily expanding. Although only part of the story, increased consumption of easily metabolized sources of energy has been an important component of the increasing prevalence of various metabolic disorders in Western society.

Potatoes, tomatoes and chocolate

When in 1598 or thereabouts, Thomas Hariot, a close friend and colleague of Sir Walter Raleigh, supervised the planting of the potatoes they had brought back from Cartagena (present-day Colombia) in the New World on Raleigh's estate in Ireland, he ushered in a change in the eating habits of Western Europe from which we have yet to recover. The *pomo dei Moro* (Moor's apple) or tomato made its appearance at around the same time, presumably being brought to Europe not long after Cortez's defeat of the Aztecs, slightly earlier, in 1521. Chocolate also makes its first appearance in Europe around this time, being imported from Mexico by the Spanish; however, its condemnation by the Catholic church as a probable aphrodisiac led to slower adoption, but probably to a greater black market than for the humble potato.

The widespread cultivation and consumption of potatoes boosted the carbohydrate content of the Northern European diet dramatically while the tomato increased the palatability of savoury foods by introducing a high glutamate source other than seaweed. Glutamate, and today its stabilized form, monosodium glutamate, stimulates our taste buds – specifically those receptors that are designed to taste 'umami' (a Japanese term loosely translated as 'deliciousness'). These exotic imports opened the door to steadily increasing demand for processed foods, relying on products that were difficult, initially at least, to grow for personal consumption, and led inexorably to the mechanization of mass food production and distribution.

So in simple terms there has been a huge shift in diet in Europe and in North America over a few hundred years with a massive increase in our intake of sugar, of refined carbohydrates and of 'novel', energy-dense foodstuffs such as potatoes, tomatoes and chocolate. The rest of the world has also been sold the means to catch up in those processes by a market-hungry, growth-led industry.

Commercial high-carbohydrate cereals such as flaked or puffed corn (the cornflake was 'invented' by W.K. Kellogg in 1894) and puffed rice taken at breakfast with milk are now commonplace, but are recent high-carbohydrate confections of the past century.

The chemist Joseph Priestley first made drinkable carbonated water in 1772. Carbonated high-sugar drinks first came into vogue as recently as 1886 when Dr John Stith Pemberton devised a sugar syrup which when added to carbonated water produced a refreshing drink – Coca-Cola®.

As humans have evolved, at a conservative estimate, over something like the past four million years, the above changes signalled a radical change in diet over a vanishingly small period of evolutionary time, prior to which a high-protein, high-fibre, low-carbohydrate and low-sugar diet had been consumed by all. The evolution of our bodies to adapt to indigenous fare has been rapidly overtaken by the evolution of the food-processing industry. This has enabled us to be exposed worldwide to an ever-changing range of foods, flavour enhancers, hormones, additives, preservatives and colourings. This is without mentioning the various pesticides, herbicides, antibiotics, organophosphates and phthalates, which come along with many of them as unwanted additional baggage.

How access to food has changed

The changes seen in the Western diet, first from hunter-gatherer to subsistence farmer and then from being self-sufficient to our current situation with most of the population divorced from obtaining food, and more and more even from making our own meals, makes us highly dependent on the manufacturing and distribution systems of a progressively more centralized food-processing industry. This industry is geared to maximizing profits, rather than ensuring the health benefits of the foods that are produced. High-profit, longer shelf-life convenience foods have for the past half-century gradually displaced fresh unprocessed foods in our everyday diets to a larger and larger extent. By pointing this out, I am not inferring malice, rather lack of appreciation of many of the factors we discuss here.

Major changes in consumption today tend to come about not due to the discovery of new exotic plants or animals. Changes today tend to be due to disasters or political misadventure. The BSE (bovine spongiform encephalopathy) ('mad cow disease') scare in the UK led to a massive drop in beef sales, Edwina Currie's comments on salmonella set UK egg sales into a tailspin, George Bush senior's Presidential comments on his dislike of broccoli did the same for American broccoli sales, and media coverage on the H5N1 'avian flu' virus has had major effects on poultry production and poultry sales across the world, however unlikely a species jump to humans of a mutated form and an ensuing worldwide flu pandemic like that of 1916 may be.

Occasionally there are positive results of political intervention – in New York City, in November 2006, the Board of Health stopped the use of trans-fats in cooking by imposing a ban on their use which otherwise would have likely continued as they are both cheaper than other fats to produce and less likely to go rancid so can be stored and used for longer.

The advertising budgets of Coca-Cola® and McDonald's for 2003 have each been estimated at some 1.4 billion dollars (Ad-Brands 2003). The advertising budget for Coca-Cola® in the UK alone that year was £27 million, dwarfing the £5 million which the British Government invested in promoting healthy eating across the board. It is little wonder that rates and costs of diet-related health problems are spiralling out of control (Lang 2003). The extent to which such economic factors are involved in how our diet is changing is often little appreciated (see Cannon 1987, 2005).

The increased availability of alcohol generates huge amounts of tax revenue. It is a goose that lays crates of golden eggs. Although seen as 'recreational' consumption and not part of the diet, alcohol has also become a progressively larger component of the Western diet. The result has been steadily increasing problems of cirrhosis and heart disease rivalling those seen in 18th century England. On ascending the British throne in 1689, William of Orange abolished tax on grain spirits to discourage the drinking of French wine with the result that cheap gin almost literally flooded the country. As caricatured in William Hogarth's famous print 'Gin Lane' of 1751, such problems became endemic through oversupply and increased ease of availability.

Supplementing the diet

There is a considerable history in the 20th century of successful supplementation programmes to address malnutrition for medical conditions such as marasmus and kwashiorkor – the so-called PEM (protein-energy malnutrition) diseases. This has typically been in 'Third World' countries where food restriction can be endemic. We are also starting to understand the effects of such conditions on the immune system and susceptibility to infection (see Schaible and Kaufmann 2007).

In contrast, despite the fact that the size of the supplement industry in the West is enormous, its effects are largely unresearched and underregulated. While the pharmaceutical industry has gone down the road of large-scale randomized controlled trials to establish efficacy and risk of medications, the supplement industry has been more closely allied to the food manufacturing businesses from which it originally emerged. This has led to markedly cheaper supplements than would otherwise be the case, but with a far weaker knowledge base than would have been the case had they gone down the pharmaceutical route. For whatever reason, despite being a multi-billion dollar industry, the use of food supplements has been caricatured as a fad bought into by the 'worried well' and of no real relevance to health. As we shall see, the evidence, although not as robust as much of the pharmaceutical literature, suggests that supplementation is far from irrelevant and can be quite the opposite.

General supplementation with minerals, vitamins and essential fatty acids has been shown to decrease challenging behaviour in various populations (for example, see Gesch et al. 2002; Hamazaki et al. 1996; Schoenthaler and Bier 2000). Anecdotally, the rates of challenging behaviour in many residential facilities for ASD have fallen when healthy eating has superseded convenience (energy-dense, high-fat and high-sugar) foods and drinks.

A number of books are now available which deal with general aspects of nutrition, behaviour and mental health (see, for example, Holford and Colson 2006; Richardson 2006a). In both the UK and the US, recent reports have highlighted the importance of diet in behaviour and mental health (Associate Parliamentary Food and Health Forum

2008; Learning and Developmental Disabilities Initiative 2008). A number of books are also available dealing with specific dietary approaches to ASD (Lewis 1999; Seroussi 1999; Seroussi and Lewis 2008). The principal flaw in the literature to date is in being overinclusive – the general books assume that everyone requires the same optimum diet and those which deal with ASD assuming that every ASD person has the same problem with casein and gluten digestion/a fatty acid deficiency/a specific vitamin deficiency/another specific dietary factor and that, therefore, everyone with an ASD should be helped by adopting the same diet. Neither conclusion is justified.

There are also books which cover a wider range of complementary and alternative medicine (CAM) therapies than are dealt with here. It is likely that many people will be using a combination of such approaches. Lisa Kurtz, a US occupational therapist, provides a useful overview of the range of such treatment approaches in her recent book (Kurtz 2008).

As nutritional aspects of foods change over time, it is helpful to have some fairly up-to-date sources of information to consult on the nutritional, mineral and vitamin content of foods. The standard text on this area is the much revised and updated *McCance and Widdowson's The Composition of Foods*, last published in 2002 (Food Standards Agency 2002). Another resource that many will find useful is *The Calorie, Carb and Fat Bible 2008* (Kellow, Costain and Walton 2008). It is far more detailed than anything comparable which could be reproduced here. It provides a basic breakdown of carbohydrate, calorie, fat, protein and fibre content of a wide range of over 22,000 foods, including those prepared and sold by the major supermarket chains, and provides a simple and accessible guide to many of the questions that someone who is implementing the Simple Restriction Diet (SRD) will need to ask. It also gives a breakdown for the menus served at many of the major fast-food and franchised coffee-shop outlets. Many of the phytonutrients present in foods are currently unclassified; however, attempts are being made to develop approaches to looking at such aspects (see, for example, Dr Joel Fuhrman's work on 'Nutrient Density': www.drfuhrman.com).

Many people with ASDs will be on concurrent medications so it is sensible to be aware of any potential effects of these, and also of the possibilities of interaction with dietary and CAM therapies. A simple guide to medications and how they work can be helpful (such as Stone and Darlington 2000 or Wilens 2008). A basic guide to how psychopharmacological interventions can be seen to work from a neuroscience perspective may be helpful (see Pliszka 2003). A number of guides deal with interactions between conventional and complementary therapies (see Fetrow and Avila 2003; Hendler and Rorvik 2001); one of the most useful remains *The A–Z Guide to Drug-Herb-Vitamin Interactions* (Lininger *et al.* 1999).

Non-food factors can also have a major influence on consumption. We know, for example, that calorie intake in children correlates with their amount of television viewing – the more television, the higher the intake – and that there is a tendency for them to eat more of the products they see advertised while viewing (Wiecha *et al.* 2006b). An unsurprising consequence is that, when not independently regulated, producers buy more food advertising space at the peak viewing times for this target audience. As children can influence parent purchasing to a large extent, food advertising is often targeted specifically at children (Lindstrom and Seybold 2004). Parents often end up buying the brightly coloured box their preschooler has seen on the television when they are on their next joint trip to the supermarket.

Sugar intake also increases with increased access to sources of refined sugars. To take two examples, more school vending machines and more frequent use of fast-food restaurants are both associated with a higher level of consumption of refined sugars by children (Wiecha *et al.* 2006a).

Autism spectrum disorders

Attempts to unravel the genetics of autism have held centre stage in recent years (see Mendelsohn and Schaefer 2008 for a brief recent review). None of us are mere genetic automata, however, and our physical and mental selves are inextricably linked (Sternberg 2001). Many factors other than genetics are important in how we develop, and the complexity of possible interactions between the gene products from the ~30,000 genes in our bodies suggests we are a long way from being able to develop a good 'bottom-up' level of understanding, working from genes to behaviour (see discussion in Noble 2006).

We now know that diet often plays an important role in gene expression (see, for example, Junien 2006), and that factors such as diet can be critical to the expression of epigenetic processes in both behavioural and physical development (Dolinoy, Weidman and Jirtle 2007).

Genetics is starting to unlock many of the mysteries of autism, and some genetic factors are important in understanding how best to help those with an ASD to overcome some of their difficulties (Abrahams and Geschwind 2008; Aitken 2008; Sykes and Lamb 2007). We are slowly piecing together the complex neurobiologies that underlie the ASDs (see Pardo and Eberhart 2007), with a wide range of processes being implicated. Our genetic understanding of the basis to ASD has developed enormously in recent years, but still has far to go. At present, it highlights what biological systems may be useful as foci for further research and intervention (the various genes involved in glutamate and lipid function, for example) and provides a basis for more efficient targeting of potentially effective treatments. There are now a number of companies offering 'off the shelf' genome screening (see, for example, www.navigenics.com; www.23andme.com; www.decodeme.com; www.knome.com). There are some reservations being voiced over the development of such commercial ventures before there is good clinical data in place to enable clear interpretations to be drawn (see Foster and Sharp 2008). Recent years have seen considerable discussion of the incorporation of sophisticated genetic testing and analysis into routine clinical healthcare (Williams 2003). It will be some time, however, before screening for the large number of specific gene differences linked to autism is likely to be available (to check on progress, a good starting point is the Autism Genetic Resource Exchange website: www.agre.org).

Despite the popularity of dietary interventions for ASD, there is surprisingly little in the way of adequate peer-reviewed clinical research, and few randomized double-blinded controlled trials exist in this area. This is partly because such research is difficult – keeping people from knowing what they are eating and drinking, then changing their diet, without them being aware, for long enough to see whether there are any effects is hard to do and is not without significant ethical problems. It is also partly because there is far less funding available for such research compared to, say, funding made available to research a new patent medication.

Unless there is a very strong incentive, food manufacturers are unlikely to rush to sponsor research on whether cutting down on or excluding their products may be beneficial. This is similar to the slow measured pace at which the tobacco industry tested the claims of effects from smoking on lung cancer, the way that automobile manufacturers welcomed research on removing lead from petrol, thus reducing engine efficiency, and the current controversies over whether industrial processes are major factors in the development of global warming.

'Evidence-based medicine' (see Sackett *et al.* 1991) is a powerful approach when evaluating the use of specific treatment approaches with specific conditions that have known biological bases. A range of techniques allow clinicians to establish how useful or how potentially harmful a given treatment is for a given condition.

Today those researching ASD tend to describe the subject area more as follows:

> Autism spectrum disorder (ASD) is a catch-all diagnosis for a set of poorly understood neurodevelopmental disorders that are clinically heterogeneous, with a spectrum of severity. (Stephan 2008, p.7)

Rather than being a clinical condition with a known biological basis, the ASDs are a spectrum of different conditions, with different aetiologies, which are likely to respond to a spectrum of different clinical approaches. It follows that one approach is unlikely to be right for all cases. Taking a single-case approach is more likely to be helpful where we know a range of treatments that work for some within the ASD population, and are not dealing with a biologically specific condition. The best treatment and management of people with ASD will come from the sub-categorization of those on the spectrum not from a search for 'the cure', from identifying what makes this individual develop autistic behaviour rather than from trying to find what causes autism.

Our understanding of the biology of autism is essentially at what could be called a 'pre-Linnaean', 'pre-Lavoisierian' or 'pre-Mendeleevian' stage. Until Linnaeus came up with a way of classifying plants our understanding of what made one plant different from another was essentially educated guesswork; the phlogiston theory of chemistry developed by Isaac Newton was unable to reconcile experimental data with theory, and many of Newton's results only started to make sense once we began to use the concept of elements (as proposed by the French chemist Anton Lavoisier); and devising the atomic table of elements made our understanding and predictions of the nature and behaviour of the elements reasonably accurate for the first time (thanks to Dmjtri Mendeleev). As it currently appears in much of the psychiatric literature, autism is a poorly understood condition with widely different patterns of presentation, associated problems and prognosis – the diagnosis itself provides little to help in saying what is likely to be best for any given individual.

A range of guides are available which review approaches to ASD treatment; however, the coverage of alternative and complementary therapies tends to be brief at best (see, for examples, Coleman 2005; Hollander and Anagnostou 2007; Tsai 2001). A number of guides for families are also available which cover all aspects of ASD; however, by their nature, they also tend to devote little time and space to coverage of dietary issues (see, for examples, Exkorn 2005; Grandin *et al.* 2006; Sicile-Kira 2006).

Do people with ASD really have gastrointestinal difficulties?

The issue of gastrointestinal (GI) involvement in ASD has been hotly debated, in large part due to the controversies surrounding the issue of a putative link between MMR (measles, mumps, rubella) vaccine and autism. If there is no link between GI problems and autism, then dietary interventions may not be all that helpful, so let's look at the evidence.

Often, GI disturbance has been attributed to faddy eating, and it is true that extreme self-imposed food restriction does occur in some cases and can have major developmental consequences (Uyanik *et al.* 2006).

There are differences in the gastrointestinal symptomology seen in an ASD group when compared either with those who have other developmental problems or to those with no such difficulties

(Valicenti-McDermott *et al.* 2006). Group differences are associated with dietary self-restriction and rejection of new foods by the ASD group when compared to the others, both of which can make dietary interventions more challenging to implement with this population.

In ASD there does not seem to be a relationship between the extent or severity of gastrointestinal symptomology and dietary intake of calories, carbohydrates, fats or protein (Levy *et al.* 2007). The lack of an association suggests that the higher rate of problems seen is more likely to be related to some biological difference rather than being purely due to nutritional factors.

A number of reasons for possible gastrointestinal disturbance being linked to ASD have been advanced.

The view of *abnormal intestinal permeability* (often called the 'leaky gut hypothesis') has been strongly advocated by several groups who claim to have found evidence of high levels of diet-derived peptides from casein and/or gluten in the urine of a high percentage of those with ASDs. The hypothesis will be discussed in the chapter dealing with CF-GF diets.

Critics of this view have made highly contrasting and essentially incompatible claims.

A group based in York, in the UK, have claimed that the presence of IAG (trans-indolyl-3-acryloylglycine – one of the gluten-derived opioids said to be involved in ASD) in the urine of those with ASD was not important as although they could detect IAG at significant levels in ASD urines (N=56), they could also find similar levels of IAG in all of the other children that they tested including non-autistic age, sex and school-matched controls (N=155) (Wright *et al.* 2005).

A second group, from Edinburgh in the UK, could not isolate opioid peptides either from the urine of 11 autistic children, from their non-autistic sibling controls, or from adult controls (Hunter *et al.* 2003). A larger study comprised urines from 68 4–11-year-old boys with autism from tertiary London and Edinburgh clinics without epileptic seizures who were not on active medications and 202 male 4–12-year-old controls (Cass *et al.* 2008). All analyses were carried out in the same laboratory as in the initial Hunter *et al.* (2003) study and again failed to establish peptiduria in either cases or controls.

In spite of the controversy over mechanism, the albeit limited data on effects of intervention with restriction diet are positive (Knivsberg *et al.* 2002; Reichelt and Knivsberg 2003). Some further limited support comes from the finding of reduced autistic symptomology in response to long-term naltrexone treatment (Cazzullo *et al.* 1999). Naltrexone is a selective opioid receptor blocking agent which would also attenuate the effects of exorphins; this would only be of relevance to the GI issue if the opioid hypothesis were correct, and may indicate the relevance of a central rather than peripheral opioid mechanism.

The issue of celiac disease, an autoimmune condition with an allergic reaction to gluten, can arise in a number of the conditions that can be comorbid with ASD such as Down syndrome and Williams syndrome (Giannotti *et al.* 2001).

In systematic reviews published in 2002 (Horvath and Perman 2002a, 2002b) Karoly Horvath and Jay Perman, gastroenterologists from Johns Hopkins Hospital in Baltimore, documents the high prevalence of gastrointestinal symptomology in the ASD population. They report detailed information from a questionnaire survey of 412 ASD children and 43 normal controls, and subsequently on interview validation with a subset (112 of their ASD children and the 44 siblings now of age to take part) (Horvath, Medeiros and Rabszlyn 2000). There were clear differences in the prevalence of gastrointestinal symptomology between their ASD cases and controls.

In an earlier case series they had shown that in ASD cases with gastro-oesophageal reflux there was a high prevalence of sleep disorders which responded to appropriate management of the reflux (Horvath *et al.* 1999).

A 2003 study reported on GI features in 103 autistic and 29 normal control subjects who were suffering from abdominal pain (Afzal *et al.* 2003). A significantly higher proportion of the autistic group was reported as having megacolon (a larger lower intestine) on rectosigmoid loading (this was seen in 54 per cent of the autistic group as opposed to 24 per cent of their controls), and they were more likely to be reported as having severe constipation (reported in 36 per cent as opposed to 10 per cent of the controls).

A survey of 500 families with ASD children (Lightdale, Siegel and Heyman 2001) found a high rate of reported GI problems.

Approximately 50 per cent had loose stools/diarrhoea, one in three suffered from abdominal pain and one in five had frequent bowel motions (three or more per day). There were no controls, however, and it is unclear how subjects were asked to take part.

A further case series report (Melmed *et al.* 2000) described 385 children attending the local ASD centre in Phoenix, Arizona, 102 unrelated controls and 48 sibling controls. They found in their ASD group that 19 per cent had diarrhoea, 19 per cent had constipation and 7 per cent alternated between the two. The combined rate for these problems was under 10 per cent in both of the control groups. How the problems were defined is not clear from the paper, but we can assume that it was the same for all three groups, indicating that such bowel problems were four and a half times more common in this ASD group.

A study of congenital anomalies found that only gastrointestinal anomalies were significantly more common in a subsequently diagnosed ASD population when compared with an age, sex and hospital-of-birth matched cohort (Wier *et al.* 2006).

Reviewing the evidence concerning GI problems in ASD (Erickson *et al.* 2005), their general conclusion was that the data was difficult to interpret if looking for an ASD-specific pattern of gastroenterological symptoms; however, it was clear that the rate of such symptoms in those with ASD was significantly higher than in the general population.

In a letter to the *Lancet* in 2003, Dr Simon Murch of the Royal Free Hospital states his opinion as a gastroenterologist treating ASD children as follows:

> This department has continued to assess children with autism on straightforward clinical grounds, since large numbers show improvement in abdominal pain and sleep disturbance if constipation, gastritis, or colonic inflammation are recognized and treated. However, not all children with autism show such response, a finding that needs further study. (Murch 2003, p.1498)

There is now acceptance of how prevalent GI problems are in the ASD population and of the need, where these are present, to manage them appropriately.

In one recent Swiss survey of a sample of 118 learning disabled adults, 43 with and 75 without comorbid PDD (PDD or pervasive developmental disorder can be taken as synonymous with ASD) (Galli-Carminati, Chauvet and Deriaz 2006), clinical reports of GI disorders were found in 48.8 per cent of the notes of the ASD group, and in 8 per cent of those with learning disability alone. The authors conclude that 'gastrointestinal disorders may be considered as a feature of PDD' (p.711).

One recent study of 24 consecutive autistic children of unknown aetiology found no clear evidence of a link between autism and the presence of intestinal inflammatory markers (nitric oxide and calprotectin) except in two of the children – one who had recently had severe *Clostridium difficile* gastrointestinal problems and one with extreme constipation (Fernell, Fagerberg and Hellstrom 2007).

So, although there is much debate and argument over why this should be the case, there is now no reasonable doubt that dietary and gastrointestinal problems are much more common findings in ASD compared with the general population, or that such problems can affect behaviour (see Erickson *et al.* 2005; Galli-Carminati *et al.* 2006; Lightdale *et al.* 2001; Melmed *et al.* 2000).

Addressing these areas can, in many cases, have a significant positive effect on behaviour and development.

In summary: Gastrointestinal problems are significantly more common in those with ASD than in others, but the nature and severity of such problems based on presenting clinical symptoms is not specific. They should be investigated on clinical merit in the individual case, and there is no reason to support the view that the comorbidity of ASD and gastrointestinal disturbance should lead to the GI problems not being investigated.

If anything, the presence of an ASD should indicate to the clinician the need to collect a clear history of this aspect of the person's development and functioning.

Diagnostic dilemmas

There is an implicit problem with the 'pick and mix' approach to behaviours that is the current basis to clinical ASD diagnosis – people with completely different behavioural profiles can all receive a diagnosis of ASD and because they have similar overall scores on the ADI-R, the ADOS or the DISCO (see Glossary) they can be entered into clinical trials as if they had the same problem, matching them with each other on some hypothetical construct of severity of autism. Clinical diagnosis is thus a very imprecise science. The basis for saying that two people have the same problem is really an act of faith that the behaviours that have been agreed upon signify a common underlying biology. It is far from clear that this view is correct or can any longer be justified.

Gradually we are coming to understand some of the different biologies which can result in ASD – the inborn error of metabolism which results in PKU, the methylation defect which results in Rett syndrome, the problem with glutamate metabolism in Fragile-X, and the problem with production of cholesterol seen in SLOS (Smith-Lemli-Opitz Syndrome), to take four. Historically, these conditions often could not be differentiated from others with ASD behaviour. Subgroups who have differences in their behaviour, prognosis and potential treatment are being divided off from others with ASD, partly on the basis of their behavioural presentation and partly on greater knowledge of their biologies.

Paradoxically, the implicit belief is maintained that, although we don't know what it is, there will turn out to be a common underlying basis to the rest of those with an ASD that will respond to a common treatment. We are now aware of over 70 genetic 'exceptions' to this common mechanism, which are implicated in a high percentage of people with ASD.

Despite extensive funding and huge amounts of effort spent in genetic profiling of large ASD populations, identification of a common genetic basis remains elusive (see Aitken 2008). It seems time to accept that there is no common genetic basis that results in ASD behaviour.

Despite the implausibility of a single causal mechanism, there is a huge incentive for many to assume there is common biological basis to the ASDs. Attempts are continually made to emphasize the similarities across ASD populations rather than looking at within-group differences (for example, see Ring *et al.* 2008).

The ASD population has now outstripped Alzheimer's disease in terms of 'market size' (Gerlai and Gerlai 2003). This is because ASD is seen as a 'cradle-to-grave' condition which is identified early in life in individuals with a normal life expectancy. If the same drug treatment were appropriate for everyone with an ASD, the financial implications for the first effective patented treatments would be enormous.

A recent review of the genetic literature came to the following conclusion:

> if different features of autism are caused by different genes, associated with different brain regions and related to different core cognitive impairments, it seems likely they will respond to different types of treatment. Abandoning the search for a single cause for a single entity of autism may also mean abandoning the search for a single 'cure' or intervention.

> (Happé, Ronald and Plomin 2006, p.1220)

The standard 'evidence-based medicine' view of treatment is that where there is an inadequate knowledge base you should err on the side of caution and recommend against 'it', whatever 'it' may be. This 'if the evidence is not robust then don't do it' view poses a slight problem when it comes to eating and drinking – don't do it until we have adequate evidence is just not a very sensible option; we all need to eat and drink.

A similar dilemma can be seen in evaluating evidence for approaches where clinicians are pretty certain about the biology – where randomized trials would put some at almost certain risk. Here studies are not done for legitimate ethical reasons – phenylalanine-free diet versus no diet in the early management of PKU is a good example (see Poustie, Wildgoose and Rutherford 1999). In reviewing the evidence for continuing this practice, the recent Cochrane review concluded:

> We were unable to find any randomized controlled studies that have assessed the effect of a low-phenylalanine diet versus no diet from diagnosis. In view of evidence from non-randomized studies, such a study would be unethical and it is recommended that low-phenylalanine diet should be commenced at the time of diagnosis.

> (Poustie et al. 1999, p.1)

In evidence-based medicine terms, this amounts to saying the evidence isn't very strong because there are no proper randomized trials, but we can't sanction trials like that so let's stick with the treatment that we think may work.

There is continuing evidence from clinical practice of the damaging effects of not treating PKU early enough. In Turkey, screening is not yet universal, and in a recent series of 146 cases (Vanli et al. 2006), all 15 of the late detected and late treated cases in this series had learning difficulties and an ASD, while none of the other 131 had such diagnoses.

Randomized controlled studies of additional treatment strategies are possible in PKU; one such study has recently been reported looking at the effects on blood PKU levels of giving large neutral amino acids (Matalon et al. 2007).

Preliminary conclusion – more research needs to be done

The general conclusion from the above is that no dietary approach will help everyone with an ASD. The evidence from reviews is usually read as showing that dietary interventions are not worth trying (Herbert, Sharp and Gaudiano 2002; Levy and Hyman 2005; Lilienfeld 2005). The flaw in this line of argument is that there are many biological differences which are sufficient to result in autism, so no particular approach would be likely to produce consistent effects without matching samples on the biological basis rather than on just the clinical diagnosis.

Exactly the same argument can be advanced for the lack of consistent evidence for beneficial effects of conventional medications such as risperidone (Jesner, Aref-Adib and Coren 2007) and SSRIs (selective serotonin reuptake inhibitors) (Posey et al. 2006) in ASD – they can be beneficial for some where warranted on clinical grounds but the current evidence does not support their widespread use in ASD.

Essentially, we are not able to identify a consistently beneficial approach to ASD because no approach will be consistently beneficial. Because there is no one biological causal basis, and a number of different factors seem to be independently capable of resulting in ASD behaviour, no one treatment will be helpful. We need to take a different approach and start from the assumption that a number of approaches may be helpful, but none will help everyone and some may prove to do nothing while others may even be damaging.

Adequate approaches to assessment and proper clinical trials of the various treatments and approaches that are being employed with the ASDs are urgently needed (Bodfish 2004; Chez, Memon and Hung *et al.* 2004; Levy and Hyman 2005). A number of large-scale studies are underway which should significantly advance our understanding of the causes of ASDs (see Szpir 2006). In the meantime, it is important to provide families who cannot afford the luxury of waiting tools to enable them to look into such approaches safely. The outcome of clinical studies which at best, assuming funding is forthcoming, are likely to be a decade off from completion, will be too late to guide families who have young children they are hoping to help now.

Although there is disagreement over which treatments are effective, one thing on which there is broad agreement is that effective treatments produce the best effects on outcome the earlier they are started (see, for example, Howlin 1998). The problem is not that there is good research that has shown dietary approaches do not work, there is just a lack of adequate evidence – absence of adequate evidence is very different from good evidence of ineffectiveness. Lack of evidence would not be a sound basis for a legal case; equally it is not a sound basis for stating that something is ineffective.

Families use dietary interventions whatever the clinical recommendations or admonitions

I can remember when the Mackarness diet, sometimes also known as the 'Stone Age Diet' (Mackarness 1976, 1980), was popular with many families whose children were referred to the Child and Adolescent Service at the Maudsley Hospital in London where I was doing my clinical training. Some families were also starting to experiment with removing milk and wheat from their children's diets, and some were giving vitamin and mineral supplements. At that time, such approaches were being used by parents in parallel with the conventional approaches they were accessing through health, education and social work.

Since that time – looking back, over 25 years – a wide range of dietary approaches have been suggested as possibly being helpful for people with ASDs. Paul Shattock in Sunderland, Karl Reichelt in Oslo, and both Karyn Seroussi and Lisa Lewis in the USA have been strong advocates for the use of casein and gluten exclusion diets. They are perhaps among the best known who have advocated this approach, though there are many others. A number of other dietary approaches such as low-carbohydrate diets, low glutamate diets, low phenylalanine diets, low oxalate diets and the Specific Carbohydrate Diet have been advocated and all appear to have produced beneficial results in some children.

Dietary and CAM (complementary and alternative medicine) approaches continue to enjoy a high level of popularity with and use by families. An Australian study of CAM use in 1993 estimated national expenditure as $621 million (Australian dollars) (MacLennan, Wilson and Taylor 1996). A 1997 survey estimated that the US equivalent expenditure was some $27 billion (Eisenberg *et al.* 1998). A recent UK survey estimated an annual expenditure of some £1.6 billion (Ernst and White 2000). Such high levels of usage are typically parallel to rather than a part of packages of care and remain largely ignored and underresearched by the clinical community (see Charman and Clare 2004).

Failure to capture information on the widespread parallel use of CAMs may have led to a critical flaw in the intervention literature to date – maybe an intensive Applied Behaviour Analysis (ABA) program/Theory of Mind training approach/social skills intervention/particular medication only works/works best/is ineffective when a particular dietary intervention is also in place, or maybe the diet is what makes the difference. Without collecting this information we will never know.

Some 'alternative' medical practitioners (for example, see Jepson, Wright and Johnson 2007; McCandless 2007; Pangborn and Baker 2005) use a variety of metabolic assessments as a basis for their interventions. Where this type of approach can be married to knowledge of specific biological mechanisms underpinning such differences it holds much promise. A variety of 'natural' approaches have been suggested for the treatment of ASDs (see Marohn 2002) and a wide range of therapies are being offered by practitioners (see Shore and Rastelli 2006).

Rather than waste time on trying methods which are not of benefit I hope that this book can take you some way towards making an informed choice based on current evidence – this may be a choice to consider such an approach or to wait for more convincing evidence to emerge – and towards being able to assess whether and how much any particular approach may be of benefit.

It is true that some complementary and alternative approaches have proven not to be beneficial and others will be proven not to be of benefit. I agree that where there is robust evidence that an approach does not work it should be actively discouraged. There has been an impressive improvement in the extent to which CAM therapists have embraced scientific approaches to evaluation of treatment (see Spencer and Jacobs 2003). A helpful overview of things to consider when evaluating the relevance of CAM treatments can be found in *Snake Oil Science: The Truth About Complementary and Alternative Medicine* (Bausell 2007). Bausell concludes that there is a significant placebo effect in many beneficial CAM treatments, and it should be remembered that such effects are equally likely to operate with conventional treatments.

Some who adopt extreme anti-CAM views appear to dismiss alternative approaches almost out of hand (see Fitzpatrick 2008 and Shapiro 2008 for recent overviews). Typically, the 'placebo effect' is cited as the reason for improvements where these are found and warnings are given about the possible negative effects of inadequately tested treatments. The flaws in pursuing this line of argument over ASD are severalfold:

1. There are no treatments, conventional or otherwise, which have shown consistent evidence of benefit, with the exception of behavioural interventions, and these are not condition specific, so discarding CAMs at present leaves a fairly bare cupboard of alternatives, and there are significant risks attached to many of the conventional treatments which are advocated.

2. The placebo effect accounts for part of the improvement seen with all therapies (for a general discussion of placebo effects, see Evans 2003); it is not a CAM-specific reason for apparent benefit or a reason to dismiss CAMs rather than anything else.

3. As ASD has multiple sufficient causes with different biologies, no specific therapy is likely to show efficacy across all ASD cases unless it would benefit everyone alike.

There is now a polarization between those who are caricatured as scaremongering conspiracy theorists for saying something may be going wrong or as snake oil salesmen for suggesting that anything might help, and those who argue that nothing can/should be done to help anyone with an ASD without all of the checks and balances of evidence-based medicine having provided an unrealistic level of proof. Perhaps unsurprisingly, the 'nothing can be done yet' lobby is aligned with the views of the pharmaceutical and food industries.

Historically we saw surprising similarities in the defence of the tobacco industry, where, for many years, the industry view, backed by numerous academics, was that the studies were not good enough to prove a link between tobacco use and cancer. The evidence that many senior scientists involved in this issue were both funded by the tobacco industry to carry out research and funded to act as expert witnesses in tobacco litigation has only recently been disclosed (see, for example, Hiilamo 2007).

Whatever the recommendations of clinicians and the quality of the research base, CAMs are currently employed by a large proportion of families where someone has an ASD. It is also true that many CAMs can interact with conventional health-based treatments (Lininger *et al.* 1999), and the parallel use of conventional medication and CAMs should always be checked with a competent and knowledgeable practitioner.

In one recent US survey of 284 ASD children, approximately 30 per cent were using CAMs (Levy *et al.* 2003). A study in one affluent US population found use of CAMs in autistic children to be some 92 per cent (Harrington *et al.* 2006). A further recent survey of 479 families found a wide range of treatments being employed – dietary interventions by 129, chelation by 32 and multiple conventional medications by many (Goin-Kochel, Myers and Mackintosh 2007). The types of CAMs used by parents themselves often predict the types of CAMs they are likely to use with their children (Yussman *et al.* 2004).

As with the interactions between colourants and additives in their effects on attention deficit hyperactivity disorder (ADHD) (McCann *et al.* 2007), analysis of such interactions is complicated. The lack of any consistent approach to assessment or monitoring of dietary factors in those with ASD both as primary treatments and during pharmaco-therapy or other forms of intervention has led to a literature on treatment effects that is patchy and difficult to interpret.

So where do we go from here?

There is still a huge amount we don't know or only poorly understand about the effects of food, food additives and contaminants – the glycation and lipoxidation of molecules, for example, which result from processes such as heat treatment, ionization and irradiation of processed foods can have strong inflammatory effects and have so far been implicated in a range of disease processes such as allergies, Alzheimer's disease, arthritis and diabetes (see Bengmark 2007). These compounds have major effects, are now common components in our diets, but they are little known to most clinicians and nutritionists. They have effects on various aspects of the immune system implicated in ASD such as TNF-alpha, interferon-gamma and interleukin-1RA (Croonenberghs *et al.* 2002).

I come from a clinical psychology background, and a strong emphasis in clinical psychology is placed on single-case methodology – not whether there is evidence from large trials that in general this or that approach will work, but whether in the individual case it does or can be predicted with a reasonable degree of likelihood to work. Can we predict with reasonable certainty whether a given approach is likely to work for me or for you, and can we then put it in place, and see whether it does? The recent emphasis on personalized genomics is similar – what is likely to be best for this person based on what makes them genetically different rather than making a best guess based on what we know from the general population.

A medical approach tends to work on the basis of probabilities, predicting, say, that there is a 60 per cent chance that this will work or that there is a 20 per cent chance of side effects. As a general way of developing services this is sound where there is adequate data – put more resources into the services that appear the safest and most likely to produce benefits. In reality, for any individual an approach either does work (a probability of success of 100 per cent) or it does not work (a probability of 0 per cent). I hope that this book will help people to work out for different approaches whether they may fall in the 0 or 100 per cent group for various different dietary strategies that seem to help at least some people with ASD.

I hope that this book provides sufficient information and resources to allow people to identify the dietary factors that may be important for them or the ASD person in their family, and, with the right help, to carry through with an appropriate programme of intervention. It provides you with the principles underlying various dietary approaches and a synthesis which gives a greater likelihood of success. This is not a dietetic text, a cookbook or a precise diet guide, and the composition of foods is always changing, and varies from country to country depending on farming practices. It should help anyone embarking on a dietary approach to understand the theory, some of the practice, and some of the potential pitfalls but it is far from the last word on the subject. This is a complex area, but is often dismissed in simplistic terms. In practice, it is relatively easy to modify diet but complicated to understand how to implement it with sufficient rigour to achieve the desired effect, and understand why it could make a difference.

> I would make three general caveats to anyone reading this book.
>
> First, if you decide to implement any of the dietary interventions that are discussed here, you should *do so only with appropriate support from someone who is knowledgeable and qualified to advise and support you in this area.* As will be apparent when you read about the specific approaches we go on to discuss, dietary approaches can be of benefit but, if not used properly, and if embarked upon without appropriate assessment, also have the potential to cause harm. This book

provides an outline and rationale for dietary approaches rather than a detailed guide covering everything you need to know and do.

Second, you should be clear that dietary intervention is not a stand-alone approach to the treatment of ASD; it is only one component of an appropriate package of care and support, and is not required for all. It may prove beneficial but is unlikely to be sufficient in and of itself. Appropriate behavioural, cognitive-behavioural, supportive and educational components are likely to be required in addition, to maximize the potential of someone who shows a positive response to dietary intervention.

Third, it is important to keep up to date with research developments. There is an explosion of work on ASD, and, although research on intervention is sparse, this will not be the case for long and many of these developments may be important for what is likely to help.

It is not because things are difficult that we do not dare; it is because we do not dare that they are difficult.

Seneca (54 BC–39 AD)

CHAPTER 2

Dietary Interventions

Why would you think of using a diet to help someone with an ASD?

A great pleasure in life is doing what people say you cannot do.

Walter Bagehot (1826–1877)

A large number of behaviours and physical features may suggest that dietary intervention could be worth trying. Go through the following list and see if some of these issues apply.

Does the person show distress to loud noises (sometimes called 'hyperacusis') or reactions to particular frequencies of sound?
Often hand driers, vacuum cleaners and lawnmowers seem particularly distressing. This problem can be linked to certain genetic conditions such as Williams syndrome (Klein *et al.* 1990). This can be a sign of problems with calcium metabolism.

Are there problems with the sleep–wake cycle?
Sleep problems are among the most commonly reported difficulties in ASD (Clements, Wing and Dunn 1986; Godbout *et al.* 2000; Oyane and Bjorvatn 2005; Richdale and Prior 1995) and are among the most disruptive to family life. A range of difficulties may be seen – difficulty getting to sleep, frequent night-waking, nightmares, night terrors, waking too early, unusual body-clock. Recent findings indicate a possible genetic basis to some differences in melatonin production.

Melatonin is the endogenous compound produced by the pineal gland in the brain, which controls the sleep–wake cycle (Melke *et al.* 2008).

Melatonin production would appear to be abnormal in a significant proportion of those with an ASD and to be associated with differences in the development of the pineal gland (Kulman *et al.* 2000; Lissoni *et al.* 2002; Tani *et al.* 2003; Tordjman *et al.* 2005).

Do they show food-related difficulties?

Things like picky eating, food avoidance, unusual food preferences – a strong preference for certain shapes, colours or textures, excessive craving for or eating of carbohydrates (e.g. biscuits, bread, cakes, muffins, potatoes, pasta). Such problems can have behavioural (see Ernsperger and Stegen-Hanson 2005; Legge 2002) and biological bases, many of which we will be going on to discuss.

Do they have excessive fluid intake?

Note if this is particularly for things like milk or artificially sweetened carbonated drinks. Excessive drinking ('hyperdipsia') can result from a number of different factors including abnormalities of the limbic system (a system in the midbrain which is involved in the control of drinking and appetite) and can also be a sign of fatty acid deficiency.

Do they have or are they suspected of having epilepsy?

Epilepsy can show itself in lots of different ways – it may be very brief periods of 'switching off' usually called 'petit mal', sudden inattention, falling in situations where the person is normally well or better coordinated, 'typical' convulsions where the person falls and jerks often with involuntary mouthing movements.

As we go on to discuss, epilepsy can respond to some of the dietary strategies which can prove effective with ASD. In a recent clinical series of 889 patients with ASDs collected by a Chicago clinic over a nine-year period (Chez *et al.* 2006), none of whom had epilepsy or a known genetic condition or clinical malformation, over 60 per cent showed evidence of epileptiform activity on ambulatory electoencephelogram (EEG) recording. In the majority, the clinical activity was over the right temporal lobe.

Do they go through phases of tiptoe walking?
There is no clear view of why toe-walking is significantly more common in ASD than in the general population. Clinically it has been linked to low circulating tryptophan levels, and there is evidence that tryptophan depletion can often initiate tiptoe walking in ASD (McDougle *et al.* 1996). Tryptophan is a dietary amino acid.

Do they have dry skin, brittle hair and nails, dandruff or 'chicken skin' on the upper arms and thighs, have they been diagnosed with asthma or atopic dermatitis, or do they have allergies, inflammatory reactions or rashes?
These can all be signs of fatty acid deficiency (Sinn 2007). There is data to suggest a link between asthma, atopic dermatitis and fatty acid deficiency (Devereux and Seaton 2005). Such features are overrepresented in ASD (Bakkaloglu *et al.* 2008).

In addition, some families use Epsom salts in the bathwater – if the skin has become dry since starting this, try adding a tablespoon of olive oil to the bathwater – always assuming that the baths appear helpful in other respects.

Are they overweight?
From chart review the prevalence of obesity is not statistically different comparing children with ASD, with ADHD and normal population controls than in the general population (Curtin *et al.* 2005).

Are they underweight?
In Asperger syndrome there is an overrepresentation of underweight individuals (Hebebrand *et al.* 1999; Sobanski *et al.* 1999). As yet, there is no clear indication of why this is the case.

Are they easily tired out or lethargic?
Various factors can lead to becoming easily tired. A number of muscular conditions are associated with ASD, such as myotonic dystrophy type 1 (Ekström *et al.* 2008). Problems with glycogen release can also cause someone to become easily fatigued; this can be seen in congenital myotonic dystrophy, which has been reported in association with ASD (Yoshimura *et al.* 1989) and can be seen in the early stages of a carbohydrate-restricted diet (Greenhaff, Gleeson and Maughan 1988).

Are they overactive/distractible/do they seem to have concentration problems?
A range of factors have been linked to these ADHD characteristics, including deficits in calcium (Oades, Daniels and Rascher 1998), zinc (Akhondzadeh, Mohammadi and Khademi 2004; Bilici *et al.* 2004), iron (Burattini *et al.* 1990; Sever *et al.* 1997) or magnesium (Kozielec and Starobrat-Hermelin 1997; Starobrat-Hermelin and Kozielec 1997), and fatty acid deficiency (Sinn 2007).

Bladder and GI symptoms – do they suffer from frequent urination, poor bladder control, pain on urination, bedwetting, constipation, diarrhoea, pains, trapped wind, large bowel movements?
Gastrointestinal symptoms and their prevalence were discussed in detail in the last section. This information need not be repeated here.

Do they show Pica?
Pica is defined as chewing on or swallowing non-food items. In general, although Pica is not uncommon in ASD, the association seems to be more with level of learning disability rather than with ASD (Swift *et al.* 1999).

Do they show evidence of self-injurious behaviour?
Many people with ASD (but far from the majority) will go through phases when they self injure. This is unlikely to be a genetic condition, although there are genetic factors which can be involved – the one that figures in many textbooks but is very rare is Lesch-Nyhan syndrome, a single gene abnormality of purine metabolism with no known treatment (see Torres and Puig 2007).

Self-injurious behaviour is one of the features of ASD which has been linked to a possible opioid system dysfunction (see Panksepp 1979). A recent animal model has also linked self-injurious behaviour to glutamate-mediated difference in brain development (Muehlmann and Devine 2008).

Conclusion

If the person being considered for possible dietary intervention has a number of the above features, there is a reasonable possibility that they may benefit from some form of dietary intervention. The next and more difficult question to address is which dietary intervention/s may be of benefit. To clarify the answer to this question, familiarizing yourself with the rest of this book should stand you in good stead.

Things to leave out which may be causing a problem

Owing, as I believe, to their chemical individuality dif-ferent human beings differ widely in their liability to individual maladies, and to some extent in the signs and symptoms which they exhibit.

Sir Archibald E. Garrod (1857–1936)

Sir Archibald E. Garrod was the first person to emphasize the impor-tance of individual differences in susceptibility – why one person is more prone to nausea/agitation/flushing in response to a food when someone else appears not to react to it at all. Prior to his work, the working assumption in medicine was that people were affected by diseases purely because they had been exposed to them – everyone would respond in the same way given the same exposure. For Garrod, however, people would react to an exposure or a disease to a greater or lesser extent dependent on their 'chemical individuality'. For many of the dietary interventions we go on to discuss, their likelihood of being beneficial depends on the biological characteristics of the person in question.

Although the notion of individual differences in biological suscep-tibility is well recognized and accepted, such differences continue to be seen as rare exceptions. The assumption is that, other than in rare instances, we can treat everyone as being the same – we will all require the same dietary intake of essential nutrients/dosage of medication. This view is much the same as saying, based on normative data, that every person should need the same size of shoes/jeans/shirt. A few clinicians have argued that the process is far more complex and that we need to be looking towards a more individually tailored approach to dietary and pharmacological management (see, for example, Williams 1998). This model is the basis to a number of current dietary approaches (D'Adamo and Whitney 2007; Wolcott and Fahey 2002), and is the basis on which compounding pharmacies operate in the USA, to provide medications and supplements as appropriate to the needs of the individual, not to the needs of Mr/Ms Average.

Some individual differences are genetic (as we will discuss, one genetic condition, Smith-Lemli-Optiz syndrome (SLOS), results in difficulties in making cholesterol and responds to cholesterol supplementation), others are environmental (an autistic child who has been breast-fed by a vegan or vegetarian mother may have much greater needs for taurine and vitamin B12, two nutrients which are virtually absent from the vegan diet). Taurine levels are severely depleted in the plasma and urine of those who adhere to a vegan diet (Laidlaw *et al.* 1988) and in the breast milk of vegan women (Rana and Sanders 1986), and the effects on the developing infant can be far greater than on the adult who will typically have chosen to adopt this type of diet at a later age.

From work on knockout taurine transporter mice, it appears that interfering with taurine uptake results in defects in skeletal muscle function (Warskulat *et al.* 2004). This suggests that if there are equivalent genetic defects in taurine receptor and/or transporter functions in humans there may be an inherited basis to differences in human taurine metabolism. Although one study has identified a transporter difference in cells cultured from human placenta, to date no *in vivo* taurine defects have been reported in man.

Part I of this book deals with the use of various dietary restrictions – limiting the intake of certain sorts of foodstuffs as a means of combating problems due to difficulties brought on by digestive differences, toxic reactions, aberrant immune responses or difficulties with clearance.

A useful introduction to many of the general issues discussed here can be found in Elizabeth Lipski's well-written and informative books on 'Digestive Wellness' (Lipski 2004, 2006).

By the way, don't get too worried if, after you get a couple of pages on, the main focus of the book seems to be on cutting down consumption of polar bear liver or poisonous fish; these are merely being used to illustrate more general ideas about possible toxic effects. Similarly with the protection given by theriacs. However sensible such recommendations could be for certain Arctic explorers, ardent sushi addicts, or ancient rulers, I don't think they are specifically relevant to someone with ASD unless they happened to fall into any of these groups.

Digestive differences

In terms of digestion, as with much else, we are not all the same. There are many differences in digestion both between individuals and between genetically different populations, some due to what we consume, some how our bodies deal with the things we eat and drink. It is important to note, therefore, that a dietary approach that has had good success in one area or with one person may not be as effective in another.

For example, difficulties with the digestion of milk sugar, also known as lactose, are common problems for many people (see Heyman 2006). They are more common in certain racial groups and are particularly common in people of Chinese origin (Yang *et al.* 2000), while much less common in Western Caucasian populations.

The Inuit of Greenland, existing on a non-processed traditional diet, appear to have certain differences in digestion such as absence of intestinal sucrase which make them better at coping on a high-protein low-carbohydrate diet than most other groups, having evolved to cope with digestion of a quasi-carnivorous diet (Ho *et al.* 1972). Such adaptations are minor in comparison with those seen in obligate carnivores and it may be that other people can survive equally well on such carbohydrate-restricted diets.

The Canadian Arctic explorer Vilhjalmur Stefansson (1879–1962) documented the fact that most Inuit appeared to live on a diet consisting largely (around 90 per cent) of sealmeat, caribou and fish, often existing for lengthy periods on nothing else – essentially, a no-carbohydrate diet. Over several decades, Stefansson developed his theories on the role of high-protein diet, meeting an initially sceptical reaction from both medical researchers and the public. To demonstrate that eating a carnivorous diet did not produce significant damaging effects,

Stefansson and a fellow explorer, Karsten Anderson, acted as subjects in an early study, published in *JAMA* (the Journal of the American Medical Association), in which they ate a 100 per cent meat diet for a lengthy period under medical observation in a New York Hospital – in Anderson's case, for a year (Lieb 1929). Both men remained perfectly healthy throughout, without taking any vitamin supplementation, fruit or vegetables. Stefansson's views are clearly laid out in his book *Not by Bread Alone* (1949). His work was the inspiration for Richard Mackarness's approach, which we discuss in the first dietary section of this book.

The English dietary researcher Hugh MacDonald Sinclair carried out a similar self-imposed 100-day-long experiment, some 50 years later in 1979. Sinclair ate largely sealmeat (delivered weekly, frozen, to the kitchen of his university halls in Oxford), together with fish and crustaceans, with no fruit or vegetables. Regular checks were carried out on a variety of physical parameters such as his blood viscosity. As with the Inuit, his clotting time lengthened as he maintained the diet. This experiment, important as it was, proved much to the annoyance of others dining at Magdalen College at the time due to the powerful and unusual smell from the sealmeat that pervaded the dining room (see Chapter 21 in Ewin 2001).

More recently it has become clear that the health benefits from this approach are to do with carbohydrate reduction, not with increased protein intake. The importance of dietary fat intake on a higher protein diet has been acknowledged for some time (Speth and Spielmann 1983).

There are many genetic differences in the ability of individuals to digest carbohydrates – the sugars and starches that form much of the typical non-Inuit diet (Swallow 2003). Differences have also been demonstrated between different ethnic populations in carbohydrate digestion (see, for example, Tsumura *et al.* 2005).

It is interesting to note that before adoption of a Western diet including processed foods with a high intake of complex carbohydrates, most hunter-gatherer societies which have been studied seem devoid of Western ailments such as stroke, ischaemic heart disease, atherosclerosis, type 2 diabetes, osteoporosis, breast cancer and obesity. Adoption of a Western diet, however, results in a steady rise in the prevalence of all of these conditions. There are obviously certain caveats here as life expectancy tends to be lower in hunter-gatherer populations and certain of these disease risks are associated with living for longer.

As food production has been industrialized, we have become steadily more dependent on a small number of food crops – a mere 17, listed in Table 2.1, now supply almost 90 per cent of all human food, with all of the major crops being carbohydrate rich.

Table 2.1 Major global arable crop tonnages per annum

	Million metric tons	% of world food production
Wheat	468	22
Maize	429	20
Rice	330	16
Barley	160	7.5
Soybean	88	4
Cane sugar	67	3
Sorghum	60	2.8
Potato	54	2.5
Oats	43	2
Cassava	41	2 (see Cyanide below)
Sweet potato	35	1.6
Beet sugar	34	1.6
Rye	29	1.4
Millet	26	1.2
Rapeseed	19	0.9
Bean (all)	14	0.7
Peanuts	13	0.6
Total	**1910**	**89.8**

(Adapted from Cordain 1999; Harlan 1992)

An overview of toxic reactions

As with general differences in digestion, toxic reactions can also be variable and complex (see Brent *et al.* 2005). Some will show major reactions to foods which are tolerated well by others. Gradual insidious exposure can acclimatize the body to a higher toxic load than could be tolerated with rapid exposure.

Taking complex but dilute mixtures of poisons, venoms and other noxious agents to ward off the effects of environmental toxins has a lengthy history. Known historically as 'theriacs', their consistency gave us the English word treacle. King Mithridates the 6th, Eupator of Pontus (132–163 BC), is reputed to have survived repeated attempts to poison him by taking a concoction known as the *'mithridatium'*, made up of 36 poisons in low doses, taken every day. After the defeat of Mithridates the 6th by the Roman legions of Pompey in 66 BC, the *mithridatium* and its closely guarded recipe was taken to Rome, gradually tested and modified, and by the time of Galen, the theriac devised by Nero's physician Andromachus, and taken daily, was a mixture of 64 ingredients.

The various *mythridatia* used by generations of Greek and Roman leaders were complex blends of poisons that led to gradual conditioning of the body to tolerate larger and larger doses of otherwise lethal substances (see Flanagan and Jones 2001). Many years later when political assassination by poison had become almost commonplace in the Renaissance Italy of the Borgias, 'Venice treacle', based on the older mithrodatia, became a popular protective and was being used well into the late 18th century (see Pain 2008).

A well-known proponent of this method of self-protection was the Russian priest Grigory Rasputin who survived poisoning with cyanide-laced cake and wine, only dying after then being shot several times and finally being chained in a trunk, dropped in the *Dnieper* river and drowned (see Moynahan 1998).

The general point here is that most humans have adapted to having regular exposure to low level toxins whose introduction is insidious. A number of recent studies have shown that such low level exposures are affecting all of us, whether Inuit, !Kung, Aborigine, subsistence farmer or supermarket shopper (CDC 2003; Houlihan *et al.* 2003; WWF 2007).

Due to their extensive use in the middle of last century, we all have significant levels of toxins in our bodies from pesticides and flame retardants that can affect brain function. In a recent study, the WWF examined samples from 155 volunteers from 13 locations around Britain, looking for 78 chemicals in blood (WWF 2003) – 12 organochlorine pesticides (including lindane and DDT), 45 polychlorinated biphenyl congeners and 21 PBDE flame retardants. All of the people who were tested were contaminated with compounds from each of these three groups. The highest concentration found was 2557 ng/g of p.p'DDE – a DDT metabolite. This is despite the fact that the use of DDT was banned in the UK over 20 years ago. Ten of the compounds were found in over 95 per cent of those tested including p.p'DDE. These findings are surprising especially in view of the virtual absence of lindane and endosulfan from the present European food chain (Fontcuberta *et al.* 2008). Similar concerns are now being raised over possible toxic problems arising from the use of organophosphate insecticides (see Shattock, Carr and Whiteley 2007).

A number of toxic compounds have therapeutic implications for treatment of clinical disorders as they operate to interfere with bodily symptoms. The use of leeches to draw blood was painless and effective due to the complex chemistry employed by the leech to both anaesthetize the donor site and prevent coagulation (see Plotkin 2000). The possible role of conatokin NMDA receptor antagonists, derived from marine cone snails, in the treatment of epilepsy is a further recent development in harnessing complex natural biochemistry (Jimenez *et al.* 2002).

Fugu

The lethal reputation of Fugu, the various types of pufferfish so enjoyed as part of Japanese sushi, is due to the presence of the compound tetrodotoxin found in the liver, gonads and skin of these fish, particularly at certain times of year. Tetrodotoxin is thought to be the product of a bacterium which only affects the fish during certain climatic conditions. This is a fast-acting neurotoxin that typically kills within four to six hours by paralysis of the respiratory muscles, through interfering with the outer pores of the sodium channels involved in nerve conduction (see Isbister and Kiernan 2005).

Preparation of Fugu to remove any tissue containing tetrodotoxin is a delicate and skilled task, and Japanese chefs need to be accredited before being allowed to prepare it. A number of deaths from tetrodotoxin poisoning are still reported every year in Japan as a direct result of eating Fugu.

The fish is banned from sale across the European Union (Regulation (EC) 853/2004 App. III Sec. VIII), and only 17 restaurants in the USA are licensed for the preparation and serving of Fugu, mostly in New York.

There is nothing to link terodotoxin exposure to ASD. It is discussed here purely as an example of one of the extreme effects of acute toxic exposure.

Vitamin A

Some substances are highly toxic in excess and need to be avoided in large amounts though these same substances may be essential at low levels.

As we have already mentioned, vitamin A depletion through self-restricted diet can result in severe visual loss (Uyanik *et al.* 2006).

The vitamin A content of polar bear liver is so high that as little as 1/3 g is at the upper limit of recommended human adult daily consumption and eating 30 g could easily prove fatal (while cod liver oil has some 600 units of vitamin A per gram, and human liver around 575 units, polar bear liver contains some 24,000–35,000 units per gram).

It has been argued that the deaths of the ill-fated balloonists in the Swedish 1897 Andrée balloon expedition to the North Pole were due to consumption of polar bear liver when they were forced to overwinter on White Island on their return journey south from the pole (for a popular account of this ill-fated expedition, see Howell and Ford 1985).

Vitamin A is biologically essential, and it has been argued that in certain cases high dose supplementation can be helpful to people with an ASD (Megson 2000). As with the polar explorers, however, such a course of treatment should not be embarked on lightly and not without appropriate medical investigation, establishing a metabolic deficiency in vitamin A, tests of liver function, and close supervision throughout.

Mercury

When the Hatter made his appearance at the mad tea party in *Alice's Adventures in Wonderland* in 1865, Charles Dodgson (aka Lewis Carroll) concatenated features which were well recognized in the milliners of his day.

This behavioural pattern was not some personality difference in people that led them to go into hatmaking. It was an effect of slow mercury accumulation resulting from the processes involved in making felt hats from fur pelts. The process was necessary to mimic the way in which beaver fur naturally coalesces and flattens due to the naturally roughened edge of the strands of fur, which produces a smooth finish. As beaver pelts became scarce from overtrapping, this process was introduced to enable other furs to be used creating a similar smooth effect. The process typically involved the use of mercurous nitrate at an early stage to roughen the hairs and enable them to mat together more easily in the subsequent felting process. Inhalation of the mercury vapour at this and subsequent stages resulted in various symptoms of mercury toxicity including coordination problems, irritability, personality change and anxiety. The changes observed in hatmakers at this time led to the term 'mad as a hatter'.

Mercuric nitrate was finally banned from use in the hat industry in 26 states of the USA on 1 December 1941. The ban was imposed because of a shortage of mercury for military use, not as a consequence on the effects seen in hatmakers.

One possibly important factor concerning mercury and ASD is that mercuric compounds can interfere with the functioning of some members of a family of factors known as aquaporins (Savage and Stroud 2007). Aquaporins are a class of compounds that form water channels in cell membranes. In animal models, aquaporin expression in the gastrointestinal system can be affected by the induction of food allergy (Yamamoto, Kuramoto and Kadowaki 2007), thus affecting water absorption in the gut wall.

MERCURY-CONTAMINATED TOXIC WASTE – MINAMATA BAY, JAPAN 1956

One of the best known toxic reactions is the tragic teratogenic effect of mercury from eating seafood poisoned with toxic effluent from Minamata Bay in Japan (Smith 1975).

What came to be known as 'Minamata disease' affected residents of Kumamoto and Minamata, two small towns about 570 miles southwest of Tokyo. Reports began to appear in 1956, with similar clinical reports emerging from ingestion of mercury-polluted seafood from a different area, at Niigata, on the Agano river, in 1965. Symptoms vary, but many have marked deformities, particularly of the limbs, often with 'flipper-like' arms and legs. When, in 1958, the Corporation switched its dumping to the Minamata river which drains into a different area past the town of Hachimon, within a few months people in this area started to present with the same symptoms as those from Kumamoto and Minamata (for an introduction to this disaster, see Kondo 2000).

A high seafood diet was felt to be implicated from an early stage, and Dr Hajime Hosokawa, an employee of the Chisso Corporation, identified mercury toxicity from residues and, more specifically, the effect of mercury dumping by the Chisso Corporation. He illustrated the problem in 1959 by demonstrating the effects of acetaldehyde poisoning of cats to senior Chisso Corporation management. The consequence was that he was restricted from carrying out further research and the Corporation withheld his results. Mercury dumping did not cease until 1968, some 12 years after the problem had been identified. The company has admitted to the dumping, between 1932 and 1968, of some 27 tons of mercury compounds into Minamata Bay, much resulting from the production of acetaldehyde and the plasticizer diotyl phthalates. Over 3000 people have been identified as suffering with Minamata disease, of whom hundreds have now died. The Japanese courts are still resolving the process of compensation for most.

MERCURY POISONING THROUGH EATING TREATED GRAIN

Treatment of grain not intended for human consumption with antifungal alkyl-mercury compounds has resulted in several documented episodes of human poisoning through eating grain from treated seed. Episodes have been reported from Iran, Iraq, Guatemala and Pakistan (see, for example, Amin-Zaki *et al.* 1974). The Iraqi incident happened due to eating bread made with grain that had been treated with a methylmercury-based fungicide; this happened in the autumn and winter of 1971–1972. Over 6500 cases were admitted to hospital, of whom 459 died. The use of such grain in the food chain was prohibited in most Western countries in the 1960s.

The amount of mercury applied to agricultural land in the form of pesticides, however, has remained extremely high. One study (Murphy and Aucott 1999) has estimated that over the period from 1921 to 1990, in New Jersey alone, some 318,000 lb of mercury has been applied to their 1,500,000 acres of cropland and golf courses, while had they been following recommended pesticide levels they would have applied between 600,000 and 1,000,000 lb.

TOXIC PHENOL WASTE SPILLAGE – DOOSAN, SOUTH KOREA, 1991

In March 1991, the Naktong River, which supplies drinking water to over 10 million families in one of the most populated areas of South Korea, was polluted with 320 tons of phenol waste that leaked from a burst underground pipe in the factory at Doosan Electro-Materials Inc. The leakage was of a highly toxic phenol residue from processes used in the manufacture of copper-laminate computer circuit boards. The company was ordered to cease production for one month. After two weeks the ban was lifted due to the effects on hundreds of other Korean industries reliant on their output. Thirteen days later, a further phenol spillage into the Naktong River from the same plant occurred. The company also admitted to earlier lower levels of phenol release into the water supply. The spillage caused a range of problems from nausea and sickness to neurological deficits. Some 12,000 individuals and 30,000 businesses filed for compensation against the Doosan Corporation. Approximately £15 million was paid in individual compensation; 700 of those filing for compensation were pregnant women, but to date no follow-up research has emerged on the infants born to those who were exposed.

At the time of the incident, the Doosan Corporation owned the Korean franchise for a range of international products including Coca-Cola®, Nescafé, and Kentucky Fried Chicken.

Phthalates

Phthalates are compounds (aromatic diesters) which have been added to PVC during manufacture which improve a variety of aspects of the resulting material, particularly improving its flexibility, strength, and temperature resistance. The resulting material can contain up to 20–40 per cent phthalates (Jaeger and Rubin 1973). Phthalates have been extensively used in the second half of the 20th century – in blood bags and PVC materials used in special care baby units, surgical, haemato-logical and intensive care units (Luban, Reis-Bahrami and Shoert 2006), in children's clothing (Pedersen and Hartmann 2004), teethers, plastic toys and preschool play equipment. A wide range of other exposures is present, from plastic flooring to various elements used in the cosmetics industry (see Dorey 2003).

In July 2005, the European Parliament voted to impose a perma-nent ban on six phthalates with carcinogenic, mutagenic and teratogenic effects that have been used to soften the plastic in many toys and childcare products. These compounds – DEHP, DBP, BBP, DINP, DIDP and DNOP – have been used for many years in toys and childcare articles which young children sucked and chewed; rubber ducks, dolls and teethers have typically been high in phthalates. There is no definite evidence that any problem has arisen; however, the 'precau-tionary principle' has been exercised given the research evidence of the effects that can arise from exposure.

In the spring of 2005, Greenpeace tested a range of toys, reporting that, among others, 'Spiderman Flip 'n Zip and Mattel's Barbie "Fashion Fever" contained high levels of harmful phthalates' (Peters 2005).

The EEC ban is on the use of these compounds in toys and other products that are likely to be mouthed by children.

Equally worrying is the use of phthalates in materials such as the PVC gloves often used during food preparation. A Japanese study (Tsumura et al. 2001) found that significant levels of food contamina-tion from DHEP in packed lunches, detected in 5 out of 16 prepared lunches examined, were almost entirely caused by the use of phthalates-containing gloves, particularly when they were sterilized with an ethanol spray.

When DEHA (Bis(2-ethylhexyl)adipate) is used in food-grade PVC film for wrapping foods like cheese, it is rapidly absorbed into cheese slices to levels that after ten days considerably exceed European Union guideline levels (Goulas *et al.* 2000).

The damaging effects of Di-2-ethylhexyl phthalate (DEHP) exposure in animal research have been known for some years (see Tickner *et al.* 2001).

Many materials used in special care nurseries for premature infants have had components made from phthalates-softened PVC. This has historically resulted in high levels of exposure to infants in special care, in particular, at a highly vulnerable period in early development. This was well known but felt to be an acceptable risk from intensive life-saving procedures which required the use of phthalates-softened PVC materials (Calafat *et al.* 2004); unfortunately, the most compromised infants received the highest levels of exposure of up to 50 times normal levels. The evidence, although limited, suggests an association between being born extremely premature and likelihood of severe developmental disabilities including autism (Halsey, Collin and Anderson 1996). To date no studies have specifically examined phthalates levels in ASD.

Lead toxicity

Lead toxicity (aka 'plumbism', 'painter's colic' or 'saturnism') has been recognized at least since 250 BC when Nicander of Colophon described anaemia and colic due to lead exposure. Our current understanding suggests that insidious low-level exposure can cause developmental problems in the foetus and young child (see Needleman 2004).

Cases of autism have been reported in association with frank lead toxicity (Accardo *et al.* 1988). Blood lead levels in children with ASD are elevated (Filipek *et al.* 1999). In one small series, 44 per cent of ASD cases (8/18) had significantly elevated levels in comparison to controls (N=10) (Cohen, Johnson and Caparulo 1976).

Children with ASD treated for lead toxicity tend to have higher lead levels than other children presenting with lead toxicity and to accumulate lead again after treatment (Shannon and Graef 1997). This could indicate re-exposure – returning to the activities that lead to the accumulation – or be due to greater retention of lead if the normal clearance pathways are not as efficient.

In this context, sources of exposure may be important.

A TELLING EXAMPLE

The RC2 Corporation withdrew large numbers of Chinese-made 'Thomas the Tank Engine' infant and toddler toys in 2007. This was because it was found that they were painted with lead-based paints. These toys had been on sale in both the USA and Europe for some considerable time. The numbers of toys withdrawn was large (some 1.5 million toys were withdrawn from sale); however, the numbers which had been sold before the problem came to light is not known and the possible effects of lead ingestion through exposure have not been adequately studied.

The strong interest in Thomas the Tank Engine shown by many with ASD is well recognized and was documented in a 2002 study by the UK National Autistic Society (see: www.myfavoritetoys.com/autism_thomas.php). There may therefore be a more insidious basis to the reported obsession with Thomas the Tank Engine seen in young children with ASD than was previously suspected.

Antimony

Antimony is a toxic metal which, as antimony trioxide, is a key constituent of many modern flame retardants used in fireproofing of materials, particularly plastics and plastic foam in mattresses (see Liepins and Pearce 1976).

Antimony is more easily accumulated in the body if there is a low level of selenium. Although antimony is relatively benign in normal circumstances, of possible importance in ASD is that cytotoxicity associated with antimony exposure is linked to abnormalities of the c-jun-kinase gene, which is found on chromosome 17 at p11.2 (Mann *et al.* 2006). This is a gene locus, which is implicated in the pathogenesis of two separate conditions linked to ASD – Smith-Magenis syndrome (Hicks *et al.* 2008) and Potocki-Lupski syndrome (Potocki *et al.* 2007). It is thus possible that in Smith-Magenis and Potocki-Lupski syndromes there may be a greater susceptibility to problems from antimony exposure.

Arsenic

Arsenic can be found in a number of foodstuffs such as edible seaweeds like Kombu, much used in Japanese cooking, and supplements such as powdered kelp which is often suggested by alternative practitioners, as a rich source of iodine, in the management of thyroid dysfunction. A case of arsenic poisoning through the use of a kelp supplement has recently been reported (Amster, Tiwary and Schenker 2007).

In 1955, 12,000 infants in Kyoto were accidentally poisoned by 'Morinaga' powdered formula milk that had become contaminated with arsenic (Ohira and Aoyama 1973). Some 131 antimony poisoning associated deaths in exposed infants were reported and a large number of lesser toxic reactions. Compared to breast-fed infants and other formula-fed infants who were not exposed to the contaminated milk, neurodevelopmental problems were elevated tenfold (see discussion in Grandjean and Landrigan 2006). Long-term follow-up of this cohort has recently been reported suggesting that exposure to some 60 mg of arsenic over several weeks was required to result in significant neurotoxicity (Dakeishi, Murata and Grandjean 2006).

On a far larger scale, arsenic poisoning has resulted from the water drawn from tubewells which were sunk extensively throughout Bangladesh in the 1960s and has had a major impact on huge numbers of the population (see Meharg 2005).

Alkylphenols

These are compounds extensively used in manufacturing processes for paper, textiles, lubricating oils, pesticides, metals and plastics. They can be found in a range of foodstuffs. Contamination is mainly from discharge from these processes (Ferrara *et al.* 2005; Guenther *et al.* 2002). Alkylphenols are endocrine disruptors and their effects have been noted in the feminization of various species of male fish in response to sewage effluent both around the UK (Peters *et al.* 2001) and in other parts of Europe (Vethaak *et al.* 2005). They are now readily detected in a range of human tissues such as umbilical cord blood and in substances such as breast milk.

Cyanide

To take another unusual but, for some, more directly relevant issue, some people with ASD show evidence of a build-up of cyanide. In terms of diet, the main significant food source is the West African staple crop cassava (Osuntokun, Monekosso and Wilson 1969). Cassava (*Manihot esculenta* Crantz) is now used much more widely in the world food supply, being used in some types of Asian and European cuisine, as well as being a staple in the West African diet. It is widely used in many other areas: in the Caribbean (principally the Dominican Republic, Jamaica, Puerto Rico, the Eastern Caribbean and Bermuda), Central America (Costa Rica and Panama), South America (Bolivia, Brazil, Colombia, Paraguay, Peru and Venezuela), many countries in Africa, and Asia (India, Indonesia and the Philippines). Although not used to any significant extent in North America or Europe, 41 million metric tonnes are produced for human consumption each year.

Almonds and the stones of certain fruit – apricots, peaches and plums, all of which contain a compound called amygdalin – can be metabolized to produce cyanide by enzymes and bacteria in the gut.

This potential problem with cassava is reported in the Nigerian literature (see Okafor 2004), but is otherwise not widely known. Other possible cyanide sources are from tobacco smoke and from the manufactured chemical form of vitamin B12 known as cyanocobalamin. Another, extremely rare dietary source of cyanide is from the cycad nut consumed by the Chamorro people on the island of Guam. Eating cycad flour, cycad nuts, and bats, which consume high amounts of the nuts themselves, may be the cause of the complex disease presentation Lytico-Bodig disease, resembling a combination of amyotrophic lateral sclerosis, Parkinson's disease and dementia seen in this population. As bat and cycad flour consumption has fallen, the rate of this neurological presentation has also declined from a rate at its highest reported of 40 per 10,000 to a rate of some 2.2 per 10,000.

Although it is a rare complication, the use of cyanocobalamin can lead to retinal damage and, with one type of visual impairment seen in association with ASD (Lebers hereditary amaurosis (LHA)), can accelerate visual loss due to the build-up of cyanide caused by the abnormal liver metabolism seen in this condition. Cyanocobalamin, an artificial vitamin, is the most readily available form of vitamin B12 in pharmacies and health food shops.

Table 2.2 lists a number of well-documented toxins and their recognized effects.

Table 2.2 Chemical toxins and their effects

Chemical group:	Alkylphenols (octylphenol, nonylphenol)
Found in:	Umbilical cord blood, breast milk
Likely effects:	Can cause immune, developmental and reproductive disorders
Chemical group:	Bisphenol A
Found in:	Umbilical cord blood, amniotic fluid, placental tissue, breast milk, adult ovaries, adult blood
Likely effects:	Can cause immune developmental and reproductive disorders
Chemical group:	Brominated flame retardants (PBDEs; TBBP-A; HBCD)
Found in:	Umbilical cord blood, breast milk, breast fat, adult blood, adult fat
Likely effects:	Can cause developmental, reproductive and nervous system disorders and cancers
Chemical group:	Organotins (dibutyltin; tributyltin; trimethyltin; triphenyltin)
Found in:	Adult blood, adult liver
Likely effects:	Can cause immune, developmental and reproductive disorders and cancers
Chemical group:	Phthalates (DEHP; DINP; DBP; BBP; DIDP and DNOP)
Found in:	Child blood and urine, adult blood and urine
Likely effects:	Can cause immune, developmental and reproductive disorders and cancers
Chemical group:	Artificial musks (musk xylene; musk ketone; AHTN; HHCB)
Found in:	Breast milk, adult blood, adult fat
Likely effects:	Can cause developmental and reproductive disorders and cancers

Abstracted and adapted from Dorey (2003).

Potentially protective factors

Selenium

Selenium was discovered in 1817 by the Swedish chemist Jacob Berzelus and named after Selene, the Greek goddess of the moon. It is an essential trace mineral that plays an important role in the clearance of heavy metals.

To date, more than 25 genetically determined human seleno-proteins have been identified (Gromer *et al.* 2005). Roles have been demonstrated in processes ranging from cancer prevention to immune function and male reproduction (Ferguson *et al.* 2005).

Selenium levels in fruit and vegetables have been falling over recent decades due to changes in farming methods depleting selenium levels in soil. As a consequence, many people are now selenium deficient. Abnormalities of selenium metabolism have been implicated in a number of clinical conditions such as Parkinson's disease, epilepsy, Alzheimer's disease and myxedematous cretinism (Schweizer *et al.* 2004).

Overactivity of selenium glutathione peroxidase is seen in autism and in several other conditions where antioxidants have been implicated, such as liver cirrhosis and multiple sclerosis (Michelson 1998).

Effects of toxic exposure from excessive ingestion of selenium, particularly through eating astralgus, are well documented, particularly in cattle who can develop a condition called 'staggers' through grazing on this plant during drought conditions – a phenomenon which has been noted at least since the early descriptions given by Marco Polo. Excess blood levels of selenium are found in people in parts of China and Venezuela (Diplock 1993).

Selenium depletion can be equally damaging and is seen in people in certain areas of China, and as soil levels are particularly low in New Zealand, supplementation is essential (Diplock 1993; Thomson and Robinson 1980). In China, deep plowing of Loess soils heavily depleted the selenium levels on crops grown in certain areas, resulting in children being born with problems such as Keshan disease, a form of childhood onset congestive heart disease linked to stomach cancer, which became increasingly common in infants born in the Keshan and Linxian regions (Gu 1983; Keshan Disease Research Group 1979). Selenium supplementation in the indigenous populations of these areas has significantly reduced the problem (Xia *et al.* 2005). A further condition, Kaschin-Beck disease, which presents as osteoarthritis, is also reported from Central China and associated with selenium depletion and in its severe, type III form is associated with severe mental retardation (Editorial Board of the Atlas of Endemic Diseases and Their Environments in the People's Republic of China 1989).

We are developing a clearer understanding of the functions of selenium in the body (see, for example, Ferguson *et al.* 2005), and a number of selenium-dependent mechanisms have been found to be dysfunctional in some individuals with ASD, with elevation of enzymatic antioxidants such as glutathione peroxidase (see James *et al.* 2004; Sogut *et al.* 2003).

Glutathione

Lower levels of glutathione are seen in childhood and are known to be particularly low in autism (see, for review, Chauhan and Chauhan 2006). There is some evidence to suggest that reduced glutathione levels can be significantly increased through the use of a readily available health food supplement, 'pycnogenol'. This is an extract from French marine pine bark. To date, however, the safety of long-term use of this substance has not been established (Dvoráková *et al.* 2006).

(Detailed discussions of antioxidant functions in human health and disease can be found in Diplock *et al.* 1998 and Papas 1999.)

Aberrant immune responses

Some people have a true allergic reaction to certain foodstuffs. Nut allergies, for example, can result in the person going into anaphylactic shock if they inadvertently eat or come into contact with even minute quantities of certain nuts (see Luyt, Dunbar and Baker 2000; Sicherer 2002). In celiac disease, a similar but less pronounced reaction to ingestion of gluten is seen. A recent meta-analysis, however, has found wide variations in reported rates of allergies dependent on the data collection methods used (Rona *et al.* 2007).

Wide ranges of immune abnormalities have been reported in ASD, particularly in the pro-inflammatory cytokines such as tumour necrosis factor alpha, the interleukin receptor antagonist IL-1RA, and inter-feron-gamma (see Croonenberghs *et al.* 2002). A recent study had found evidence of abnormalities of sulphur amino acid metabolism, critical to immune system functioning and particularly in the control of oxidative stress reactions (Suh *et al.* 2008).

Difficulties with body clearance

For some, the problem can be one of inadequate clearance of com-pounds from the body that are metabolized and excreted effectively by others.

The current controversy over potential effects of mercury build-up (with various hypothesized sources – from seafood and dental amalgam to mercury-based vaccine preservatives) hinges for its validity on the view that certain individuals have defects in the clearance mechanisms for heavy metals. This is different from the issue of exposure to toxic levels of mercury affecting everyone as in the Minamata situation discussed above.

If present, such differences could be due to defects in the produc-tion or function of aspects of the body's heavy metal clearance systems such as compounds called metallothioneins (see Aschner *et al.* 2006).

The limited information to date has not shown differences in immune responses comparing lymphocyte samples from autistic probands on the Autism Genetic Resource Exchange (AGRE) database to sibling controls; however, larger and more adequate studies are still needed (Walker, Segal and Aschner 2006). Information on hair levels of mercury comparing autistic infants to controls is suggestive of possible excretion problems, but also requires extension and replica-tion (Holmes, Blaxill and Haley 2003). There have been suggestions, based on urinary metallothionein levels, that differences in metal clear-ance are due to defects in the metallothionein pathways (Nataf *et al.* 2006). This is an open review of a self-selected series, however, and further research is required before these findings could be seen as robust. Some preliminary data from a comparative study casts some doubt over the validity of the original data (Shaw 2008).

A similar area of individual difference that may result in difficulties is the abnormality of a gene called PON1 and its association with ASD (see D'Amelio *et al.* 2005). The paraoxonase 1 (PON1) gene is involved in the ability of the body to metabolize and excrete organophosphates. In the United States, where organophosphate exposure is higher due to more intense farming methods, there appears to be a link between differences in PON1 and likelihood of ASD, whereas in Europe this does not appear to be the case. This may be an example of what is known as a diathesis-stress effect – where you need both the genetic propensity to the problem together with a critical level of exposure, with the combination of the two leading to the problem.

If a person has recently undergone extensive medical treatment involving surgery/blood transfusion/saline drips or has been in neonatal or adult intensive care, it may be sensible to have phthalate levels checked. Typically this is only likely to be a problem if there is ongoing exposure.

If a person has high levels of exposure to passive smoking, is or was a smoker, consumes cassava on a regular basis, has hepatic (liver) problems, consumes cyanocobalamin (one particular widely available form of vitamin B12) as a vitamin supplement, or shows evidence of retinal degeneration, it may be sensible to check for possible cyanide toxicity.

If a person has a tendency to suck or chew on toys – especially Thomas the Tank Engine – sucks on his or her hands when dirty, chews or sucks on clothes or bedding, it may be sensible to check for lead and antimony toxicity.

If there is evidence of elevated levels of heavy metals, it may be sensible to check selenium levels and for problems with clearance pathways.

PART II

DIETS FOR PEOPLE WITH ASDS

CHAPTER 3

So, What Diets Are Currently Used with ASDs and Why?

A range of diets have been recommended to help people with ASD, and the area has often been steeped in controversy – most recently over whether the opioid/leaky gut theory makes sense.

Remember that there is a difference between whether something works and an understanding of why it works. This is a contrast which was drawn by the English philosopher Gilbert Ryle. He talked about the difference between 'knowing how' and 'knowing that' (Ryle 1949). You can ski without understanding how it happens or being able to explain it ('knowing how' without 'knowing that'), you can know the theory behind skiing and not be able to ski ('knowing that' but not 'knowing how'), you may be able to do both ('knowing how' and 'knowing that'), or, more typically (in my case at least), you may be unable to ski but not able to work out why you can't (not knowing how or that).

I have laboured this point a little, because it is important to grasp. Much of the criticism of dietary approaches is based on testing theories about why a given approach might work and not on clinical research into benefit. This amounts to saying 'this can't work' (we may not have looked to see but on principle we believe it can't) rather than 'this doesn't work, and here is the evidence which proves this beyond reasonable doubt'.

If the wrong theory is being tested, we arrive at the wrong conclusions. William Thompson (Lord Kelvin) 'proved' that evolution was impossible because on his calculations our sun was about 30 million years old while Darwin was estimating that evolution on earth involved processes which he thought would take hundreds of millions of years. For Thompson, evolution was impossible as the earth wasn't old enough for it to have taken place. Thompson was drawing a flawed conclusion; the various proofs that a heavier than air craft could not fly or an iron boat could not float today suffer from a similar lack of factual support and seem ludicrous in retrospect. Testing or proposing theories is all very well; what we really need to know is whether something works in practice, and whether it works in the situations that we are interested in.

If we briefly consider casein-free gluten-free (CF-GF) diets, there is (albeit limited) clinical research but this broadly supports improvements being linked to dietary restriction for some at least (see, for example, Millward *et al.* 2008). Research has challenged the theory (the knowing how) component of this approach – whether, if there is an effect, it could be due to a more highly permeable gut wall coupled with incomplete digestion of casein and gluten, leaving opioid residues which go on to affect brain function. Testing the model has resulted in contradictory failures to replicate. There are claims that everyone produces such opioids in urine so the finding is non-specific (Wright *et al.* 2005), and other claims that these exogenous opioids are impossible to find (Cass *et al.* 2008; Hunter *et al.* 2003). These are not findings that say *whether* CF-GF diets work; they address one model of why they could work assuming that they did – they test out one theory about the mechanism, not whether the diet actually works. The outcome of these researches is thus a possible need to come up with a different theory for why those who improve on a CF-GF diet appear to do so, rather than concluding that, as the theoretical basis proposed is questionable, therefore there could be no benefit.

It seems odd that the CANDAA (CAN Diet Affect Autism) study, an attempt to test out the question of whether such diets do indeed work, has had great difficulty attracting funding. This is especially odd since the MRC research review (MRC 2001) identified this as one of a number of research priorities. If systematic research demonstrated that CF-GF diets were effective, it would be important to identify why – what factor or factors led to the improvement; if, however, such research were to demonstrate a lack of effects, trying to establish why would be wasteful of resources.

Given that for many of the diets that are advocated there is a limited evidence base, I have provided a systematic review of the evidence base (knowing that – does it appear to work for some) and the theory (knowing how – what are the theories concerning why it might work) that underpin the principal dietary approaches advocated to date.

Certain common factors, which may be involved in the beneficial effects reported by different approaches, emerge from this overview. In addition, a range of potential difficulties is identified with many of the approaches that are often not fully discussed in the literature to date.

This overview is provided to enable people who are using any of these approaches with benefit to see whether there are things they need to be aware of or might be able to improve on. It should also help those who have run into difficulties to identify possible reasons for these.

Part III of the book provides details of the Simple Restriction Diet, an approach which draws on the common principles which cut across the diets in Part II that have shown benefit, and provides ways of minimizing the potential difficulties seen in the other approaches that have been described.

CHAPTER 4

The Mackarness (Low-Carbohydrate, High-Protein) Diet

No diet will remove all the fat from your body because
the brain is entirely fat. Without a brain, you might
look good, but all you could do is run for public office.

George Bernard Shaw

The Mackarness or 'Stone Age' diet was an early systematic attempt to
alter body metabolism as a way of addressing various physical and
mental health problems. The diet (Mackarness 1976) was based on the
clinical experience of Dr Richard Mackarness, a UK general practitioner who subsequently trained in psychiatry and moved into working on
dietary exclusion, establishing the first UK allergy and obesity clinic,
and worked extensively with patients who had different forms of
mental illness (see Mackarness 1959, 1976, 1980). A number of other
clinicians have continued and extended from his original work (for
example, Hodson 1992). His first book, *Eat Fat and Grow Slim*, appeared
in 1958 and sold over 1.5 million copies. As a high-protein, low-
carbohydrate dietary approach, it preceded the first book produced by
Robert Atkins – *Dr Atkins' Diet Revolution* (Atkins and Herwood 1972),
and the wide range of similar high-protein diets which have appeared
since, such as the Paleo diet (Cordain 2002), Neanderthin (Audette and
Gilchrist 1995) and the X Factor diet (Kenton 2002). None of these
approaches has made specific claims for benefit in the treatment of
ASD. A fairly detailed review of a range of low-carbohydrate diets can
be found in Kauffman (2004), and a detailed historical review of much

of the research on low-carbohydrate diets in weight management can be found in Taubes (2007).

Similar dietary regimes have been used for much of recorded time to improve bodily function, and are essentially the pre-agrarian, hunter-gatherer subsistence diets of many societies even today (see Cordain *et al.* 2002a; Milton 2000). Athletes in ancient Greece training for the original Olympics some two millennia ago were encouraged to adopt a diet high in fresh meat and low in vegetables.

The earliest clearly detailed low-carbohydrate diet can be found in the '*Physiologie du gout, ou Méditations de Gastronomie Transcendante; ouvrage théorique, historique et à l'ordre du jour, dédié aux Gastronomes parisiens, par un Professeur, membre de plusieurs sociétés littéraires et savantes*' (*The Physiology of Taste*) by the French judge, epicure and gastronome Jean Anthelme Brillat-Savarin (1825).

Brillat-Savarin had grasped that bread, cakes, pasta, and potatoes caused overweight and suggested a diet, which I paraphrase as follows:

> At breakfast barley-bread is a necessity, and take chocolate or strong café au lait rather than regular coffee.
>
> Barley-bread in place of bread made with refined flour. Soups made with julienne of green vegetables, cabbage and roots, but not soup au pain, pates or purees.
>
> At dinner, any starter except rice aux volailles or the crust of pates. For the second course, avoid everything farinacious, but eat roasts, salads, and herbacious vegetables. For sweet, fruits of all kinds, confitures. After dinner, coffee, liqueurs, tea and punch.

In the context of the diet consumed by most in his day, which was high in bread, pasta, high-carbohydrate vegetables and sugar, Brillat-Savarin's observations and recommendations would have constituted a large drop in carbohydrate intake, and despite a few 'mistakes' – barley bread is not much different from the wheat breads it was being recommended to replace, and hot chocolate was not an improvement on coffee – would have been seen as a major change in eating habits in a period where corpulence was seen as an occupational hazard and sign of success.

In 1863 in England, William Banting produced his *Letter on Corpulence Addressed to the Public*. This pamphlet is often cited as the first book on dieting. Banting was a carpenter and undertaker, famed in his day for making the coffin for the funeral of the Duke of Wellington. He was 1.52 m (5'5") tall, and at his heaviest he weighed 92 kg. His principal complaint that led to his dieting was not of his being overweight, but of deafness. His problem with hearing was caused, according to one of his doctors, by a narrowing of the ear canal resulting from his obesity. Banting consulted the London physician William Harvey, who had recently attended a lecture in Paris by the French physiologist Claude Bernard on the effects of liver function in diabetes (see Bernard 1865). Under Harvey's direction, Banting successfully lost 19 kg by adhering to a diet that was high in protein, with a small amount of fruit and vegetables, dry toast, tea and not inconsiderable amounts of alcohol. He excluded bread, milk products, sugar, beer, and root vegetables. Banting's pamphlet on his diet was hugely popular, selling in tens of thousands worldwide and running to several editions. The popularity of his diet led to the term 'Banting' for dieting to reduce weight being widely adopted (it is still the term for dieting used in Sweden to this day).

The Mackarness approach had three main principles:

1. That there are different metabolic types, and it was important to recognize the metabolic type for any individual:

   the 'constant-weight always-slim' type,

   and

   the 'fatten-easily' type.

   The closest recent parallel to this view is in the *Eat Right for Your Type* diet (D'Adamo and Whitney 2002) and the more recent *GenoType Diet* (D'Adamo and Whitney 2007) advocated by Peter D'Adamo.

2. He suggested that in the fatten-easily type, there was a metabolic defect in the ability to metabolize carbohydrate, resulting in easy weight gain on a high-carbohydrate diet. Although it was unknown to Mackarness, there is now evidence of metabolic defects in carbohydrate metabolism that would have this effect (see Swallow 2003).

3. He further proposed that problems with diet, weight control and digestion have a sound evolutionary basis – *Homo sapiens* evolved as hunter-gatherers to digest and make maximal use of a high-protein low refined carbohydrate diet.

We have evolved as a species to cope with a hunter-gatherer diet in a gradual process over several million years. We have not evolved biologically at a sufficient rate to cope with the dietary changes imposed by our move from this diet to the high-carbohydrate, cereal and root crop, milk product and refined sugar diet which has emerged out of our recent development of agrarian culture and animal domestication over the past 10,000 years. A useful articulation of this general argument, developed for a different purpose, can be found in Peter Gluckman and Mark Hanson's excellent little books *The Fetal Matrix: Evolution, Development and Disease* (Gluckman and Hanson 2005) and *Mismatch: Why Our World No Longer Fits Our Bodies* (Gluckman and Hanson 2006). They have developed the view that much modern disease (diabetes, heart disease and obesity in particular) is a consequence of our developing as individuals using a genetic programme which was evolved to cope with a pleistocene environment, where often foods were either in very short supply or abundant. They argue that the ontogenic programme of the foetus is tuned *in utero* by placental exposures to maternal diet and stressors. A more general treatment of evolutionary concepts as applied to human disease can be found in Nesse and Williams' excellent little book: *Evolution and Healing* (Nesse and Williams 1994).

There is good evidence that the mechanisms involved in fat storage are highly conserved (they are little changed across species), being conserved from bacteria such as *Saccharomyces cerevisiae* to humans (Kadereit *et al.* 2008).

The view that high-protein or meat-only diets were the likely fare of our paleolithic ancestors and would result in positive effects on health and fitness have been advanced by various authors including Blake Donaldson, a New York cardiologist (Donaldson 1960). Alfred Pennington, while researching obesity in staff working for DuPont, came to a similar conclusion that carbohydrate is readily converted to fat while protein has a lesser effect on weight gain and that carbohydrate restriction would lead to weight loss (Pennington 1953a). His high-protein non-calorie-restricted diet was successful in reducing weight in many staff that adopted it (Pennington 1953b). Most recently, both the 'Neanderthin' diet (Audette and Gilchrist 1995) and the 'Paleo' diet (Cordain 2002) have developed very similar theoretical and practical approaches to diet and have proven popular in the USA for weight control, for athletic training and for the management of a range of clinical disorders.

There is ongoing debate over the precise nature of and variations across paleolithic diets, but a general acceptance that such diets were very different to the current Western ones both in content and in their effect on body physiology (Eaton and Eaton 2000). The archaeological evidence from sites such as Jerf-el Ahmar in modern-day Syria suggest that the domestication of grains such as einkorn and emmer wheat can be dated to around the 9th–10th millennium BC (see discussion in Jones 2007).

There is now strong evidence that adoption of a high refined carbohydrate Western diet is associated with increased rates of what have come to be known as the 'diseases of civilization', principally from the study of their rapid emergence in hunter-gatherer societies which have become Westernized and adopted a high-carbohydrate, low-protein diet. T.L. Cleave, who was a prominent British surgeon, wrote a highly influential book, *The Saccharine Disease*, on the negative health effects of refined carbohydrates such as white flour and sugar. He claimed, based on an extensive review of the literature, that the introduction of such foods to the diet of a population was followed within 20 years by a large increase in reported rates of problems such as diabetes, heart disease, gastrointestinal problems, and dental caries (Cleave 1974). It could, of course, be argued that such dietary changes may also be paralleled by improved access to medical services and closer monitoring for such diseases.

In parallel with increased intake of refined carbohydrate there was a drop in protein intake. There was also a change in the relative levels of omega-3 and omega-6 oils in the animals and fish being consumed. These changes were brought about through increasing domestication and progressively more intensive farming methods. There is an increasing problem with grain-based feeds being used in the intensive rearing of cattle, sheep and pigs, and in fish and crustacean farming.

When cattle were grass reared in large fields and then walked to market their lean meat had high levels of omega-3 and low levels of omega-6. These levels were in very much the sorts of proportions seen in wild animals such as antelope, deer and bison. The gradual move to grain rearing of cattle in pens coupled with heavy use of hormones, antibiotics and growth promoters, together with limited exercise has resulted in a very different picture (Cordain *et al.* 2002b), with higher omega-6 and lower omega-3 levels. In the meat of grain-fed cattle, there is two to three times the level of saturated fat compared to game meat, while there is three to four times less omega-3, where grass-fed cattle are intermediate between the two.

A useful overview of the beneficial effects of sourcing and consuming grass-fed rather than grain-fed meats can be found in Jo Robinson's book, *Pasture Perfect: The Far-Reaching Benefits of Choosing Meat, Eggs, and Dairy Products from Grass-Fed Animals* (Robinson 2004), and links to the scientific literature in this area can be found through the Eatwild website: www.eatwild.com.

There is a reasonable body of evidence for our having evolved to digest lean red meat low in saturated fats as a primary energy source. Modern farming methods have diverged the meat we obtain from that historical picture (Mann 2000).

What are the different types of dietary fats and why is this important?

There are three main types of fats that come from our normal diet – saturated fats, monounsaturated fats and polyunsaturated fats (see Figure 4.1 and Table 4.1). A fourth group, trans-fats, and their more recent successor interesterified fats (Sundram, Karupaiah and Hayes 2007) are artificially modified fats produced to improve the shelf-life and texture of foods. Trans-fats have been used in baking and catering because of their longer shelf-lives and reduced tendency to becoming rancid.

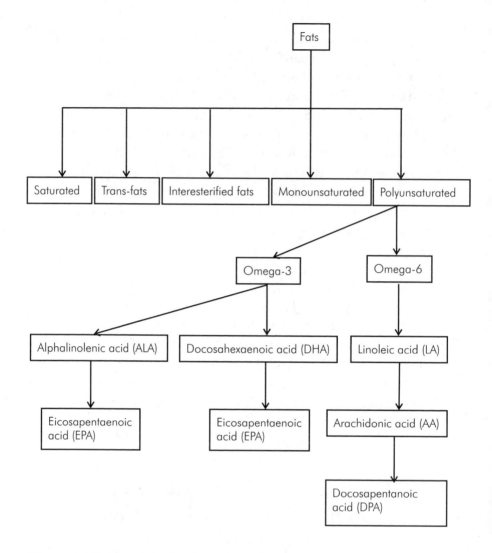

Figure 4.1 Fats and the basic pathway for PUFA degradation

The negative health effects of trans- and interesterified fats come from increasing levels of low density lipoprotein, a known risk factor for the development of both cardiovascular disease and type 2 diabetes. It is the omega-3 – ALA, DHA and EPA – that convey the greatest health benefits.

Table 4.1 Examples of fat sources in diet

Saturated fats	Monounsaturated fats	Polyunsaturated fats	
		Omega-3	Omega-6
Butter	Olive oil	Oily fish	Sunflower oil
Cream	Canola oil	Lean red meat	Safflower oil
Fatty meats	Avocado	Walnuts	Sesame oil
Chicken skin	Almonds	Pecans	Corn oil
Coconut oil	Cashews	Green leafy vegetables	Bread
Palm oil	Hazelnuts	Canola oil	Cereals
Biscuits, muffins, cakes, pastries		Omega-3 rich eggs	

Most fats are a combination of compounds called triglycerides. Triglycerides consist of a mixture of three fatty acids together with glycerol. They are broken down into these constituent elements in the intestine and absorbed as fatty acids and glycerol into the cells lining the gut wall where they recombine. Only the glycerol component of triglycerides can be converted into an energy source (glucose) that can be used by the brain. Excess glycerol is stored in the liver and released by glycogen at times when the body requires additional energy.

There is increasing interest in the role certain aquaporin channels, and their controlling genes, aquaporin-7 and aquaporin-9, play in this process of glycerol release and transport. These specific aquaporins allow glycerol to move through cell membranes and are implicated in type 2 diabetes, obesity and various other metabolic conditions (Hibuse *et al.* 2005; Wintour and Henry 2006).

In general, methods of farming have major effects on the nutritional content of the foods produced. A free-ranging Greek hen which pecks at vegetation like purslane will produce eggs with a roughly tenfold higher level of omega-3 compared to a battery-farmed corn-fed unsupplemented US hen (Simopoulos and Salem 1989).

Among the best natural omega-3 sources are 'oily' fish, and, in particular, anchovy, sardines, mackerel, salmon and tuna (Young and

Conquer 2005). Game meats such as venison are also rich natural sources of omega-3. Many foods are now enriched with omega-3 oils including some hens' eggs, margarines, milk and breads (see Young and Conquer 2005).

Why are differences in omega-3 and omega-6 levels important?

Higher levels of omega-6 oils such as arachidonic acid increase the levels of prostaglandin E_2 and leucotriene B_4 which are produced. These are pro-inflammatory molecules that will result in exacerbation of conditions with an autoimmune component.

In contrast, higher levels of omega-3 such as eicosapentaenoic acid (EPA) increase the levels of prostaglandin E_3 and leucotriene B_3 that reduce inflammation.

The differences in the production of pro-inflammatory compounds from omega-6 or 'soothing' compounds from omega-3 are important in a range of clinical conditions including rheumatoid arthritis, diabetes, and cardiac problems. The evidence to date also suggests that omega-3 can play an important role in ASDs and related conditions (see Richardson 2006a, 2006b).

EPA is important in the conversion of prostaglandin E_2 to thromboxane B_2 in the endoplasmic reticulum. These are produced from arachidonic acid. EPA is therefore important in the metabolic clearance of pro-inflammatory compounds produced from omega-6 (see Figure 4.2).

Thromboxanes are important in a range of processes: blood clotting, blood vessel constriction, and in the role of white blood cells in controlling inflammation. Leukotrienes are important in inflammatory reactions and in lung function. Prostaglandins are important factors in gastric and kidney function, blood clotting and blood vessel integrity and inflammatory responses to infection (see Agency for Healthcare Research and Quality 2004).

Omega-6 pathway

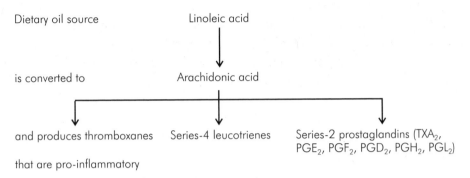

Omega-3 pathway

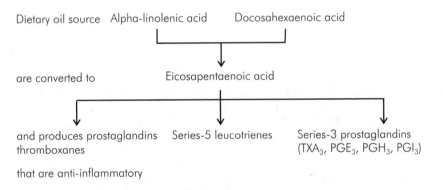

Figure 4.2 A simple diagram of PUFA metabolism

Alpha-linolenic acid is derived from plant sources such as flaxseed while docosahexaenoic acid is animal derived as is most eicosapentaenoic acid in the non-vegetarian/vegan diet.

I am labouring the omega-3/omega-6 issue because of the differences that have resulted from changes in farming methods. As we have discussed, increased use of grains in fattening domestic animals has resulted in a change in the fatty acid balance in red meats and in many farmed fish. This has fundamentally changed the likely benefits from merely adopting a Mackarness-type diet as described in many publications on high-protein low-carbohydrate diets. Today, a far more thoughtful approach is required when trying to adopt a healthy diet.

The adoption of a high-protein diet which is also high in saturated fats is potentially damaging, particularly to cardiac function in individuals who are already at elevated coronary risk (Fleming 2000), and often the amounts of saturated fat intake are excessive in people who adopt a low-carbohydrate diet – it is important to take proper dietetic advice and to limit intake of fats such as butter, cream and saturated oils, while elevating intake of monounsaturated and omega-3 oils.

A range of other factors such as perceived stress also increase the production of pro-inflammatory cytokines for which omega-6 provides the biochemical substrates (Glaser *et al.* 1999).

A recent study from Case Western Reserve University in Cleveland examining autopsy brain tissue from five autistic and five control brains demonstrated consistent findings of abnormal oxidation of lipids in the autistic samples suggesting an abnormal pattern of oxidative stress in these cases (Evans *et al.* 2008).

What is the Mackarness diet?

Essentially the Mackarness diet was one of the first systematic low-carbohydrate diet plans. For Mackarness, who drew heavily on the work of Stefansson and Cleave, many of the health and weight problems of modern man arose due to an inability to evolve as a species quickly enough to keep pace with the shift from a hunter-gatherer to an agrarian lifestyle. This shift resulted in problems stemming from increasing reliance on a diet rich in foods such as grains, sugar, cow's milk, yeast and soy in place of the hunter-gatherer diet which was diverse but relatively rich in meat, wildfowl, fish, local fruits, simple vegetables and roots. The aim of the diet was not simply to lose weight, although this usually is part of the result, but to reduce the likelihood of medical conditions such as type 2 diabetes, cardiovascular and gastrointestinal problems, and to reduce the prevalence of mental health concerns such as anxiety, depression and schizophrenia.

The theory is inherently plausible – no doubt we have evolved to be able to digest and utilize the foods which are in our natural environment, and it is equally true that over 99 per cent of this evolutionary process took place while we stuck to a hunter-gatherer form of subsistence. It thus seems likely that there may be many things that we have difficulty in digesting or may even digest too easily, in part at least because they did not form a part of our historical diet.

There may be regional/ethnic differences in metabolism which lead to differences in diet – it would be sensible, for example, that groups who have evolved to eat predominantly meat (such as the Inuit) would have evolved with more efficient digestion of meat proteins, and for those whose habitat is rich in varied fruits and vegetables to be more efficient at surviving on a vegetarian diet.

What does it claim to do?

The diet claims to reduce the load on the individual by substituting a more 'ecologically relevant' diet based on foodstuffs that we evolved to digest effectively.

The problems in achieving this come when trying to extrapolate from the archaeological hypotheses concerning tool use to an accurate estimate of paleolithic diet and from this to current diet. The theory may be correct, but it is quite non-specific in terms of what it entails.

What is the evidence?

There have been no single-case or controlled research studies on the Mackarness diet. What exist are Mackarness's descriptions of clinical cases and the publications of others who have adopted similar approaches in their clinical practice.

More recently there have been a number of systematic studies of the effects of high-protein, low-carbohydrate diets on a variety of biological parameters such as cardiovascular and renal function in the general population. In the main, these have been carried out because of concerns over possible health risks from the Atkins diet. These provide evidence of the safety of this general approach but do not give evidence of the likelihood of benefit in ASD.

Ketogenics

Ketogenic diets induce the body to use fat rather than carbohydrate for energy and have been in use for almost a century (see Wilder 1921).

Interestingly, one reason for possible success on the Mackarness diet and of other high-protein, low-carbohydrate diets may prove to be the same as the reason for beneficial effects of the ketogenic diet which is used in the dietary control of epilepsy (see Gaby 2007; Kossoff 2004; Tallian, Nahita and Tsao 1998). The earliest 'ketogenic' diets did not involve the use of high protein intake but starvation, where the body also shifts to using body fat for energy in response to extreme food restriction (see discussion in Pratt 1928).

Both cutting carbohydrate and limiting food intake per se result in the body falling back on its own energy stores – by breaking down stores of body fat and glucagon from the liver, with the resultant release and excretion of ketones in urine.

To support the possibility of a common underlying mechanism, we will discuss the results of studies of low-carbohydrate diet in epilepsy, and of ketogenic diet in Rett syndrome and in ASD.

There is preliminary evidence from two published studies, both from the same clinical group at Johns Hopkins School of Medicine in Baltimore, for a modified Atkins diet being beneficial in epilepsy (Kossoff *et al.* 2003, 2007).

There is also some preliminary evidence for beneficial effects of a ketogenic diet in the management of children with Rett syndrome (Haas *et al.* 1986) and with children who have ASD (Evangeliou *et al.* 2003). The results of these studies are tentative, and the studies did not include measures of change in factors such as EEG, but they warrant further investigation.

Evangeliou and colleagues worked with 30 ASD children. Seven did not tolerate the diet; however, of the 23 who did, 18 (60%) showed some degree of improvement on the CARS (Childhood Autism Rating Scale) which was rated as significant in two cases, 'average' in eight and minor in eight. The best results were noted in two children whose initial ASD symptomology was mild. Both of these children improved to the extent that, coincident with their diet, they were able to transfer from special educational placements to mainstream schooling.

Essentially a ketogenic diet is a high-fat diet that results in ketone bodies being given off in urine (acetone, acetoacetic acid and hydroxybutyric acid). The diet which has had some reported success in ASD is the John Radcliffe diet, a less restrictive diet than the traditional ketogenic diet in which daily food intake is balanced as follows: 30 per cent of energy from medium-chain triglycerides, 30 per cent from fresh dairy cream, 11 per cent from saturated fat, 19 per cent from carbohydrates, and 10 per cent from protein. This produces similar changes in body metabolism but is more palatable and easier to get children to adhere to than the original ketogenic diet which is significantly higher in saturated fats (see Figure 4.3).

There have been a small number of reported cardiac complications in pediatric epilepsy patients maintained on traditional ketogenic diets. This had originally been thought to be a consequence of selenium deficiency, which can itself predispose to cardiovascular problems (Chee *et al.* 1998; Neve 1996); however, several cases have since been reported in children with normal selenium levels (Best *et al.* 2000).

There is now a significant body of research into the ways in which ketogenic diets appear to modify metabolism (Gasior, Rogawski and Hartman 2006; Hartman *et al.* 2007), and on clinical conditions in which it can be of benefit. Two conditions are of particular interest here – mutations in the monocarboxylate transporter gene MCT1 which is involved in the movement of lactate, pyruvate and ketones across cell membranes in various body systems. The gene for MCT1 has been mapped to 1p13.2-p12, an area which has also been identified as a strong linkage marker for ASD (Auranen *et al.* 2002). The second condition is glucose transporter 1 deficiency syndrome in which a defect in the normal mechanism by which glucose is taken up by the brain malfunctions, resulting in epilepsy, developmental delay and motor problems. This disorder has not as yet been reported in individuals with ASD, but many of the presenting features seem similar, and beneficial results are being reported from ketogenic diets (Klepper *et al.* 2004).

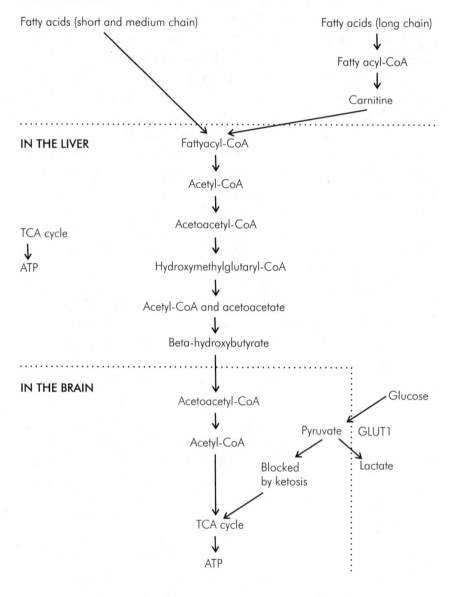

Figure 4.3 The biology of the ketogenic diet

The various gene defects responsible for this condition have been found at 1p35-31.3 (Klepper and Leiendecker 2007).

Mitochondrial respiratory chain disorders are also important here for several reasons. First, they appear to be more common in ASDs than was previously realised (Oliveira *et al.* 2007). Second, they are associated with a regressive pattern of presentation which is not otherwise typical (Poling *et al.* 2006). Most importantly, ketogenic diet has been reported as a safe and effective treatment for the otherwise intractable seizures reported in many such mitochondrial disorders (Kang *et al.* 2007).

It is well recognized that the breath of someone in ketosis can be quite strong smelling – this is typically the effect of acetone which produces a smell not unlike that of pear drops. Acetone can be further metabolized to produce small amounts of isopropanol with the result that someone who is on a low carbohydrate diet could trigger a breathalyser when tested (Jones and Rossner 2007).

A large randomized controlled trial of ketogenic diet in children with poorly controlled epilepsy, who were having at least daily seizures, has been published (Neal *et al.* 2008). All of the children enrolled in the study had achieved only limited fit control with two separate anticonvulsants and all had severe epilepsy. The study involved 145 subjects in total. Of the 73 allocated to the ketogenic dietary intervention, 65 were treated; of these, 54 provided adequate data for final analysis compared with 49 of the 72 selected controls – there was a significant dropout rate in both groups. After three months, those who were maintained on dietary intervention showed a 62 per cent reduction in seizures on average (ranging from a 50 to a 74 per cent drop). In contrast, those in the control group showed an average increase to 136.9 per cent of their baseline seizure frequency (105–169 per cent). As the baseline seizure rate was lower in the intervention than the control group and there should really have been no effect of being in the control group, the results are far from perfect; however, they do show a strong beneficial effect of ketogenic diet on seizure control. To date only the results of a three month follow-up have been reported. This is the largest and most convincing study to date on the ketogenic diet across a wide range of epilepsies, and strengthens the evidence for positive treatment effects. The principal reported side effects of the diet were constipation (in 18), vomiting and tiredness (each in 13), hunger (in 12), diarrhoea (in seven) and abdominal pain (in five).

Is there evidence of possible problems on low-carbohydrate, high-protein diets?

A number of authorities have suggested potential problems with such low-carbohydrate, high-protein diets (for example, see Bilsborough and Crowe 2003; Denke 2001), citing evidence for a range of potential and actual problems such as:

- *Heart arrhythmias*: fatty acid elevation can result from ketosis, and artificial elevation of fatty acid levels by infusion in animal models can increase arrhythmias (Soloff 1970) – this is a hypothetical risk and has not been reported clinically.

- *Impaired heart muscle contraction* – again in an animal model, perfusion of isolated rat heart with a ketone (acetoacetate) markedly and rapidly reduced contractile ability (Russell and Taegtmeyer 1991) – again this is a theoretical not a reported risk.

- *Osteoporosis* is a proven risk from ketogenic diet due to calcium loss (Sampath *et al.* 2007).

- *Development of kidney stones (nephrolithiasis)* is also a proven risk due to increased calcium excretion (Sampath *et al.* 2007).

- *Increased risk of colorectal cancer* – there is evidence for a protective effect of both increased fruit and increased vegetable intake on risk of colorectal cancer, and for increased red meat intake being associated with a slight increased risk (Sandhu, White and McPherson 2001). Both effects could be secondary to other factors such as differences between the groups studied in their vitamin intake or intake of dietary fibre.

- *Impairment of physical activity* – carbohydrate restriction reduces glycogen availability in muscle. In the person who is not physically active, this results in faster onset of fatigue and tiredness during exercise (Greenhaff *et al.* 1987a, 1987b, 1988). Acute exercise increases triglyceride synthesis in muscle, reducing fatty acid and glycerol levels (Schenk and Horowitz 2007), thus increasing ketosis to provide glucose from dietary fats and adipose stores and preventing insulin resistance.

- *Negative cognitive effects* – short-term effects on executive functions have been reported (Wing, Vazquez and Ryan 1995).

- *Optic neuropathy* – can result from low thiamine (vitamin B1) intake (Hoyt and Billson 1977). A possible effect of this diet if not avoided by appropriate supplementation.

- *Increased cortisol* in offspring of women who adhere to a high-protein, low-carbohydrate diet during later pregnancy (Herrick *et al.* 2003).

These can all be linked, in theory at least, to long-term restriction of carbohydrates in the diet.

The effects on exercise tolerance (Schenk and Horowitz 2007) suggest that a systematic programme of physical exercise (such as Cooper 1985) should be adopted in parallel with dietary restriction of carbohydrates in order to accelerate fat metabolism.

A further possible complicating factor can arise in children who have type 1 diabetes. A recent survey identified ASD as being present in 0.9 per cent of 984 children attending a Toronto diabetes clinic (Freeman, Roberts and Daneman 2005). This suggests that diabetes can co-occur with autism but not at a significantly higher rate than in the general population, so almost one in 100 ASD people are likely to have complications related to diabetic sugar control.

A condition known as 'diabetic ketoacidosis' is a frequent and potentially fatal complication of type 1 diabetes (Wallace and Matthews 2004); a major emphasis in diabetic control has been placed on the avoidance of elevated ketone levels.

The specific ketone that is elevated with poor diabetic control is β-hydroxybutyrate, which is not measured by the normal ketostrip urine testing method which has been advocated for monitoring ketogenesis on low-carbohydrate diets (this method identifies some ketones such as acetoacetate but not β-hydroxybutyrate) (see Goldstein *et al.* 1995). Where diabetes is suspected, blood testing is required to exclude ketone issues before proceeding. A positive finding would not necessarily preclude the use of a low-carbohydrate diet, and indeed some clinicians have been using this approach for many years as it stabilizes blood sugar levels, but this would have to be carefully monitored and adjusted by a clinician experienced in this approach (see Bernstein 2005, 2007).

Ketoacidosis and hypoglycaemia are potential complications of a strict ketogenic diet and such possible complications need to be closely monitored (Sankar and Sotero de Menezes 1999), as does dehydration – typically there is a reduction in fluid intake on a strict ketogenic diet, and hyperlipidaemia (Nordli 2002).

Recently, there has been increasing interest in the possible control of type 2 diabetes on low-carbohydrate diets (see Accurso *et al.* 2008).

A high-protein diet which has restricted fat has a separate set of problems – consuming more than 40 per cent of daily energy from protein can result in 'rabbit starvation' which causes gastric upset. It is described as potentially fatal by Vilhjalmur Stefansson (1944), but the suggestion is anecdotal and based on reports of trappers who were thought to have died from eating rabbit and elk which were in poor condition and low in body fat (see Speth and Spielmann 1983 for discussion).

Used as normally advised, this type of diet will result in weight loss. It should be remembered that this is typically due to a drop in calorie intake and it is more difficult to maintain calorie intake on a high-protein diet as the person feels full more quickly. But, remember, most of the studies were of its use where the intention was to lose weight. It is important to keep a careful check on weight compared to centile charts and to get regular weight checks to ensure that the approach is agreeing with the person using it. It is now reasonably well established that a low-carbohydrate, high-protein, high-fat diet is the most effective method of weight loss, but to the surprise of many also seems to have the most favourable metabolic effects on factors like low and high density lipoprotein, cholesterol and triglyceride levels, percentage body fat, waist–hip ratio, fasting insulin and glucose levels, and blood pressure (Gardner *et al.* 2007).

If considering adopting a high-protein, low-carbohydrate diet, it would be important to take appropriate supplements of calcium, thiamine (vitamin B1), a bioavailable form of iron, and to have regular checks on ketone levels in urine and of liver function as a minimum. Appropriate supplement dosages would depend on the person's age, sex and build.

Ketone tests are simple to have done and are regularly used in testing those with diabetes. Ketones can be tested for in both blood and urine. Blood tests are more reliable, but urine testing is reasonably accurate, can be self-administered, and is simpler, cheaper and less invasive to carry out.

A number of factors other than ketosis will affect ketone levels, in particular medications, such as levodopa (Darwish and Furman 1977) and valproic acid (Olson, Handler and Thurman 1986), a high intake of vitamin C (ascorbic acid), dehydration (Collett-Solberg 2001) and pregnancy (Gin *et al.* 2006).

Is there counter-evidence that low-carbohydrate, high-protein diets are less effective?

A systematic review on how effective and how safe low-carbohydrate diets are for weight loss found no consistent evidence of problems, and no link between the level of carbohydrate intake and the extent of reported weight loss (Bravata *et al.* 2003). The main predictors of weight loss were reduced calorie intake and length of time the diet was adhered to. Weight can be maintained on a low-carbohydrate diet assuming a good calorie intake is maintained. As far as weight loss is concerned, there is no evidence for greater positive or negative effects from low-carbohydrate, high-protein diets than for other approaches. The problem with most of the studies that have been carried out is that they are short term – typically six months to three years, so no long-term outcome data is available. The longer-term cohort studies of cardiac risk tend to look at relative levels of dietary intake and not at significant dietary changes likely or known to induce ketosis.

As far as ASD is concerned, there is consistent though limited evidence that approaches which result in elevated ketone excretion produce benefit, as all approaches that restrict carbohydrates can do, and only limited evidence that non-ketogenic dietary approaches are of any benefit. The exceptions are in certain subgroups where specific dietary regimes are required, as in those with certain specific inborn errors of metabolism such as methylmalonic acidaemia or hyperphenylalaninaemia. There is no reason to assume that any of the potential problems which can occur from adhering to a low-carbohydrate diet for weight loss are less likely to occur in someone with an ASD and appropriate monitoring and correction of any such problems is as important as in someone without an ASD.

In summary

The Mackarness diet has theoretical support and makes some intuitive sense. The theory does not make specific predictions concerning what should and should not be consumed, however, and there is no adequate research evidence for effects of using this or the other high-protein, low-carbohydrate diets in the management of ASD.

Many of the more recent versions of the high-protein low-carbohydrate diet are far more explicit in their dietary recommendations (see the Bibliography in the Resources section for a range of such approaches, listed in chronological order).

The one study of the Atkins diet in ASD resulted in some degree of improvement in 78 per cent of those who adhered to the diet (23/30). This suggests that it may be a worthwhile approach to investigate; however, appropriate supplementation is important, together with clear support and guidance on maintaining adequate caloric essential vitamin and essential mineral intake.

What is the relevance today?

There has been continuing controversy over the role of low-carbohydrate diets, in part because of the increased intake of dietary fats typically entailed – with particular reference being drawn to the potential for increasing the likelihood of cardiac problems, colon and stomach cancer. Surprisingly, adherence to such diets, in the short term at least, appears to affect weight control beneficially but without increasing plasma cholesterol (see Cassady *et al.* 2007).

The idea of a link between health problems and cholesterol levels comes from early research by the US public health pioneer Ancel Keys. His work on cholesterol intake in different countries and the apparent association with cardiac problems is known to many through his popular books *Eat Well and Stay Well* (Keys 1959) and *How to Eat Well and Stay Well the Mediterranean Way* (Keys and Keys 1975), and remembered by the US troops who saw action in the Second World War for his invention of 'K Rations'.

A helpful recent review of factors such as cholesterol in cardiovascular disease and the more recent recognition of the importance of omega-3 can be found in a book by the American science journalist Susan Allport (2006). *The Omega-3 Life Program* (Ratnesar 2002) is a useful little book on the practical aspects of addressing omega-3 deficiencies in a range of clinical conditions including diabetes and heart conditions which provides a useful mix of science, information on omega content of different foods, shopping and dietary advice.

For most, dietary sources of omega-3 are preferable to taking supplements. Where supplements are used, several factors need to be taken into account:

- Ensure that the supplement has adequate EPA (eicosapentaenoic acid) and DHA (docosahexaenoic acid) levels, the two most important omega-3 oils.

- Use a supplement which has vitamin E added to it as this prevents oxidation of omega-3s.

- Do not use a supplement with additional omega-6 as this has pro-inflammatory effects.

- Use a supplement with an enteric coating as this protects the supplement from being broken down before reaching the small intestine, enabling more to be successfully absorbed.

- Avoid supplements that have added vitamin A or vitamin D as these could cause problems with toxicity if used regularly.

Fish oil supplements should not be taken, or only with medical recommendation, in cases of:

- diabetes
- asthma
- blood clotting disorders or
- where any medication that has a blood thinning effect such as aspirin, warfarin or heparin is being taken.

The relevance of protein and fat metabolism to mental health was championed for many years by Dr David Horrobin, whose excellent book *The Madness of Adam and Eve* (2001) makes a strong general case for the role of essential fatty acids in cell membrane function, and for abnormalities of lipid function in cell membranes being an important and neglected aspect of a range of conditions such as schizophrenia and autism. Horrobin suggests that it is differences in these fundamental structural components of cells that can affect the ways in which neurotransmitters operate, and that the psychopharmacological approach to modifying serotonin and dopamine is operating at a level which is unlikely to affect improvement if factors such as membrane function are not also addressed.

A number of ASD conditions have associated problems with cholesterol metabolism – Smith-Lemli-Opitz syndrome (SLOS) (Aneja and Tierney 2008; Tierney, Nwokoro and Kelley 2000; Tierney *et al.* 2001), for example, is a defect in the gene coding for 3 beta-hydroxysteroid Delta7-reductase. This defect results in a lack of cholesterol production. SLOS responds to cholesterol supplementation. A useful discussion of the link between SLOS and autism with a clinical case presentation can be found in a paper by Bukelis *et al.* (2007) which deals with the effects of lowered cholesterol levels on myelination, serotonin, GABA and glutamate transporter function, and oxytocin receptors, differences in all of which are implicated in ASD.

Based on recent epidemiological data, SLOS may be the most common genetic condition associated with ASD. It has a high population prevalence, at least in parts of northern Europe, something which was unrecognized until recently (Ciara *et al.* 2006). (For a recent review of the biology of SLOS see Yu and Patel 2005.)

More generally, some 19 per cent of ASD cases in a recent study had significantly lowered cholesterol levels compared to the rest of the population (Tierney *et al.* 2006). This suggests that a significant subgroup of those with an ASD may have abnormalities of essential fatty acid metabolism.

Resources

Books

A huge number of books and resources on low-carbohydrate dieting are available. Almost all are aimed at weight control; however, some are focused on health issues such as controlling sugar level in diabetes. I provide a list of some of the better-known publications in this area as a stand-alone appendix separate from the main bibliography.

Inevitably for a model which flies in the face of conventional dietary wisdom there are many who dissent from the utility of the high-protein, low-carbohydrate approach as used for weight management.

For a reasonable flavour of the alternative position, that any such approaches are obviously evidence of dubious and dangerous 'quackery', see Michael Greger (Greger 2005), and www.atkinsexposed.org for discussions of possible problems with adhering to low-carbohydrate diets.

Similar anti-low-carbohydrate diet information can be obtained from the Physicians Committee for Responsible Medicine website at: www.pcrm.org. This site is predominantly focused on vegan and vegetarian lifestyle information but is a useful source of information on research studies dealing with possible problems with low-carbohydrate diets.

Some further reservations concerning the Atkins approach from a more balanced nutritional perspective can be found at: www.drfuhrman.com in the section entitled 'The Atkins Cancer Revolution'.

There are a number of useful overviews of ketogenic diets in the management of epilepsy:

Freeman, J.M., Kossoff, E., Freeman, J.B. and Kelly, M.T. (2007) *The Ketogenic Diet: A Treatment for Children and Others with Epilepsy* (4th edn). Demos Medical Publishing: New York.
Snyder, D.A. (2007) *Keto Kid: Helping Your Child Succeed on the Ketogenic Diet.* Demos Medical Publishing: New York.

Websites

www.autismcounselor.com/autism_diet.html

www.atkins.com is the official site for the Atkins Nutritionals Inc. – primarily a site dealing with achieving and maintaining weight loss.

www.weightlossresources.co.uk/lostart.htm is a UK site with several more critical evaluations of high-protein, low-carbohydrate diet plans; again, this is a weight-loss site.

www.ourcivilisation.com/fat links to an online version of the original Mackarness *Eat Fat and Grow Slim* book.

www.thedaisygarland.org.uk/thedaisygarland.html is a useful and well laid out website to help families of children with learning problems and intractable epilepsy learn about and implement a ketogenic diet.

CHAPTER 5

The Feingold Diet

What is it?

This is an additive elimination approach developed in the USA by Dr Ben F. Feingold initially as a treatment for hyperactive behaviour (Feingold 1975; Feingold and Feingold 1979). It has been used extensively to help people with ASD, particularly in those individuals who have problems with overactivity and concentration. Although the media coverage focused on particular colourings, specifically on the effects of tartrazine (E102), a synthetic lemon-coloured azo food dye derived from coal tar, the approach advocated by Feingold was significantly more complex than this.

The key to the original Feingold approach was the removal of three types of food additives:

1. Synthetic colourings – artificial colour, certified colour, synthetic colour, colour added. FD and C No., or by name, such as tartrazine.

2. Synthetic flavours – the only flavour listed by name is vanillin.

3. Preservatives –

   ○ BHA – buylated hydroxyanisole

   ○ BHT – butylated hydroxytoluene – vitamin A palmitate, low-fat skimmed milk, shortening, lard, beef and chicken fat, oil, gum base

   ○ TBHQ – tertiary butylhydroquinone.

and one group of artificial sweeteners:

4. aspartame, neotame, alitame.

Since the original diet was developed, our knowledge and the use of a wide range of additives, preservatives and unwanted toxins has burgeoned and there are now a vast array of potentially developmentally damaging compounds to which we are all regularly exposed.

Those who use the Feingold approach continue to refine their interventions based on evidence for interactive effects between food additives. Evidence for effects of food additives and colourants from well-conducted trials is not in short supply (Lau *et al.* 2006; McCann *et al.* 2007).

In concluding a discussion of the McCann *et al.* (2007) paper in *AAP Grand Rounds*, the monthly journal of the American Academy of Pediatrics, Dr Alison Schonwald concludes as follows:

> the overall findings of the study are clear and require that even we skeptics, who have long doubted parental claims of the effects of various foods on the behavior of their children, admit we might have been wrong. (Schonwald 2008, p.17)

In the UK, the Foods Standards Agency has announced the phasing out of a number of food colourants (Sunset yellow (E110), Quinoline yellow (E104), Carmoisine (E122), Allura red (E129), Tartrazine (E102) and Ponceau 4R (E124)) as a precautionary measure, based on this recent research.

The support materials provided by the Feingold Association for families in the USA and Canada include detailed listings of foods and provide information on a number of additives, which although not part of the Feingold program per se, can be helpful to those wishing to restrict intake of foods such as corn-based sweeteners, monosodium glutamate, calcium propionate, desulfiting agents, benzoates and nitrates/nitrites either as part of a Feingold approach or a broader dietary approach.

Having removed the above colourings, flavourings, preservatives and sweeteners, the next stage is to remove all natural and artificial salicylates. Salicylates are 'aspirin-like' compounds found in a range of foodstuffs such as citrus fruit.

If restriction of the diet results in improvements, then the next stage is to reintroduce them systematically, testing for sensitivity until specific foods or food groups that produce a negative reaction are identified, so that a diet excluding those specific foodstuffs can be constructed.

It is recommended that natural and artificial salicylates are removed as far as possible from the diet (see Table 5.1). A list of sources is provided by the Feingold Association based on a list provided in one of his papers (Feingold 1982).

Table 5.1 Significant dietary sources of salicylates

Almonds	Apples	Apricots
Aspirin	Benoral	Berries (all)
Cherries	Cloves	Coffee
Currants	Cucumbers	Grapefruit
Grapes	Lemon	Lime
Nectarines	Oil of Wintergreen	Oranges
Peaches	Peppers	Plums
Pomelos	Prunes	Raisins
Tangerines	Tea	Tomatoes

(Benoral is a soluble aspirin-paracetamol ester)

Temporarily remove natural and artificial salicylates:

- Test for dietary sensitivities by food reintroduction.

- Assess what amount can be tolerated. (If there is a reaction, is a reduced amount tolerated?)

- Begin with the fruit or food which the person misses most.

- If there is a reaction, tolerance may develop over time so remove the food from the diet but repeat the exercise periodically.

- If there are sulfation problems try to keep phenol intake low to take the stress off phenol sulfotransferase and the sulfation system, or try other strategies described in the low phenol section.

The Feingold diet can also be individualized to allow for additional sensitivities through the following:

- Use the approach in parallel with a CF-GF, SCD or other diet discussed here to try to obtain additive effects.

- Reduce dietary glutamate (see the section on the GARD diet).

- Test for and treat specific food allergies if found.

- Remove dietary benzoates: sodium benzoate, benzoic acid preservative, or naturally occurring in foods.

- Keep to a diet low in sulfites and foods treated with sulfur dioxide: residue in corn syrup, cornstarch, and dried fruit (e.g. sulfured apricots), wine, raw apple, raw potatoes to prevent browning.

- Lower fluoride exposure – consider fitting a water filtration system. A number of researchers feel fluoride may trigger central nervous system (CNS), learning and behaviour problems (Masters and Coplan 1999; Mullenix *et al.* 1995; Varner *et al.* 1998). Fluorides are found in fluoride supplements, drinking water and dental products. Silicofluorides are now used in 90 per cent of US water supplies. This may increase absorption of lead. Commercial silicofluorides may contain traces of arsenic, and other heavy metals. Blood of children from silicofluoride-treated communities can be significantly higher in lead (Coplan *et al.* 2007).

The emphasis on salicylates is similar to that which we find on the low phenol diet (see Chapter 11). Salicylates are similar in molecular structure to phenols and are thought to have similar metabolic effects.

Many of the issues discussed under toxic reactions in Chapter 2 would be considered under such an extended Feingold approach.

What does it claim to do?

Proponents of the Feingold diet claim that it can reduce hyperactivity, impulsivity, compulsions, and emotional concerns, improve attention, reduce seizures, improve toileting, and can improve sleep.

What is the evidence?

Studies which have systematically addressed the issue of effects of food colourings and preservatives using randomized controlled trials have demonstrated that in some cases there is clear evidence of behavioural reaction to colourings and preservatives (for example, Bateman *et al.* 2004; Rowe 1988). The Feingold approach per se has no strong support in more than a small percentage of cases for its use in ASD or in ADHD for which it was originally proposed (see Krummel, Seligson and Guthrie 1996).

The general approach to dietary restriction and systematically testing by challenge to establish possible sensitivities has much to commend it.

The acknowledgement of the effects of toxicants, additives and colourants is an important aspect of trying to ensure as good a diet as possible. The lack of adequate systematic research on additive or multiplicative effects of these factors makes this no easy task (Cory-Slechta *et al.* 2004), and as factors such as stress can also complicate the issues both before birth (Hougaard and Hansen 2007), and after (see Cory-Slechta *et al.* 2004, 2008), no easy answers are likely to emerge quickly.

The variety of potential factors covered in the first part of this book demonstrates that the adoption of this type of approach, examining possible effects of additives and toxic exposures, may be an important component of any dietary intervention and would be a worthwhile component to build into a dietary analysis.

Does it work?

There is no systematic research on the Feingold diet with ASD. Parent reports to the Autism Research Institute on their standardized rating scale for effects of biomedical interventions found the following ratings from 758 who responded concerning the Feingold approach: worse (0%), no change (45%), better (55%) (N=96).

Is there any evidence of possible problems?

As long as you are able to ensure adequate supplies of 'additive-free' foods that are low in natural salicylates, there are no suspected problems with adhering to a Feingold dietary regime. A significant proportion of parents who have adopted the approach claim that it has been beneficial for their child, but there is no systematic research evidence either to support or refute its utility.

An ever-expanding range of pollutants, including pesticide and fertilizer residues, glycated and lipoxidated compounds (Bengmark 2007), growth promoters, hormones, antibiotics and other compounds such as alkylphenols (WWF 2007) are now in the food chain. Any of these may have significant developmental or behavioural effects. There are also a range of exposures to compounds such as deoxynivalenol, a fungal metabolite found in cereals which is toxic in animal studies and found extensively in the human diet, but where there is no human safety data (it was identified in the urine specimens of 297/300 adult subjects in a recent study; see Turner *et al.* 2008). Obviously, these factors will have an effect on all of the dietary interventions we are discussing; however, the increasing complexity of such toxic factors in recent years is likely to have more of a negative effect on an approach which aims to curb exposure as its principal mode of action. What is required is a 'Feingold+' approach that tries to minimize exposure to all of the above.

Most of these are now factors to which we are all chronically exposed and by which we are all probably affected (see discussion in

Chapter 2 – Shattock *et al.* 2007; WWF 2003). We are now past the point of no return with regard to the possibility of conducting adequate randomized controlled trials of the effects of such exposures in real-world environments.

The 'Failsafe' diet

A similar approach, known as 'the Failsafe diet', was developed in Australia by Sue Dengate; see *Fed Up: Understanding How Food Affects Your Child and What You Can Do About It* (Dengate 2003). This is based on the exclusion diet approach developed at the Allergy Unit of the Royal Prince Alfred Hospital in Sydney, Australia (see www.cs.nsw.gov.au/rpa/allergy).

Resources

Further information

The Feingold Association of the United States
554 East Main Street
Suite 301
Riverhead, NY 11901
USA
Tel: +1 800 321 3287 (US only)
Tel: +1 631 369 9340 (Eastern Time)
Fax: +1 631 369 2988
Email: help@feingold.org
Website: www.feingold.org/index.html

A helpful introduction to the 'Failsafe' approach can be downloaded from www.fedupwithfoodadditives.info/extras/Failsafebooklet.htm.

Further information on Failsafe can be obtained through the Australian Food Intolerance Network, at: www.fedup.com.au.

CHAPTER 6

The Specific Carbohydrate Diet

What is it?

The Specific Carbohydrate Diet (SCD) was developed by a New York paediatrician, Sidney V. Haas (1870–1964), who pioneered dietary treatments for celiac disease. He had noted that removal of most carbohydrates from the diet led to symptomatic improvement and that many celiacs could tolerate banana flour and plantain meal as sources of carbohydrate (Haas 1924). He subsequently discovered that a variety of vegetable and fruit sources of carbohydrate could be safely introduced into the diet without any adverse reaction. This work was done well before we began to understand the immunological basis to celiac disease. His work culminated in the publication of *The Management of Celiac Disease* in 1951 together with his son (Haas and Haas 1951). A discussion of the development of dietary treatment for celiac disease can be found in Gottschall 1997.

What does it claim to do?

The SCD, or variations of it, have been used for almost a century in the management of a range of conditions including inflammatory bowel diseases, epilepsy and ASD. The main focus of treatment is to repair and restore the gastrointestinal system. The theory is that improvement is achieved by correcting bacterial and yeast imbalances and overgrowths, and reducing gut inflammation. 'Correct the GI tract and the rest will fall into place.' The diet has been used by a significant number of ASD individuals and families to address gastrointestinal problems.

The diet is complex and prescriptive with no gluten, no grains, and no flours (except nut and banana flours). Parents often go on to experiment with this diet having found there are benefits from a casein- and gluten-free diet but wishing to see whether this more stringent approach can provide additional benefit.

Children who progress to the SCD from a CFGF diet begin with an introductory diet for the first two to five days.

This introductory diet allows only carbohydrates that do not feed intestinal microbes, only fresh or frozen meats, poultry, fish, eggs, nuts, if at the start the person has diarrhoea then fruits and vegetables are introduced slowly after diarrhoea subsides, home-made goat's milk yogurt fermented for at least 24 hours to break down all of the casein and lactose, and, as appropriate, a number of approved supplements and medications which may include probiotics, Super Nu-Thera with P5P, cod liver oil, vitamin C, magnesium glycinate, Enzyme Complete, DPP-IV and melatonin.

SCD diet protocol

The simple carbohydrates that are allowed are in a range of fruits, in honey, some limited vegetables and nuts, and in slowly fermented home-made yogurt (where the lactose has been converted to glucose and galactose).

The protocol allows simple (monosaccharide) sugars – these are sugars that are single molecules (glucose, fructose, galactose) and are found in honey, ripe fruits, and some vegetables.

Complex (disaccharide) sugars are not allowed on the SCD. These are sugars that consist of two sugar molecules that are broken down by enzymes into monosaccharides. For example, the enzyme lactase breaks lactose down into two simple sugars – glucose and galactose.

Complex sugars are sucrose, lactose, maltose, isomaltose (found in table sugar), milk products, molasses, brown sugar, maple syrup.

Starches (polysaccharides) that are chains of sugars are not allowed (amylose, amylopectin, grains, corn, rice and potatoes).

As the principal group of clients considered for this approach are individuals with a range of GI problems, these should be thoroughly assessed before beginning.

Are there practical difficulties with following the SCD?

It is very restrictive and difficult to follow the SCD if you are unclear about the theory. You need to familiarize yourself with the ideas before trying to implement the diet as, otherwise, it is easy to make mistakes.

The introductory diet relies heavily on chicken and eggs (this may pose practical problems if there are food allergies/hypersensitivities). As nuts and nut flours are extensively used, this may elevate serum copper levels. This is possibly problematic as elevated copper is a distinctive feature of ASD. There is some evidence that people with ASD have lowered levels of ceruloplasmin, the compound that binds copper and removes it from plasma (Chauhan *et al.* 2004), and that this is critically related to oxidative stress in ASD (Chauhan and Chauhan 2006). As elevation can be linked to challenging behaviour (Walsh *et al.* 1997), and also to clinical disorders such as Wilson's disease where the elevated copper levels can damage both liver and the CNS (Das and Ray 2006), it is important that this aspect of a SCD is carefully monitored. There is some variation in this finding across other studies, with some groups failing to find similar group differences (Torsdottir *et al.* 2005).

What is the evidence?

There are no published studies on the use of the SCD. What has been published is detailed information on how to implement the approach (see Gottschall 2004). The principal interest in this approach preceded the development of the scientific method in clinical medicine. It was adopted for use in the management of celiac disease early in the 20th century.

Is there any evidence of possible problems?

The restriction of carbohydrates again is likely to restrict caloric intake, reduce intake of thiamine (vitamin B1) which has potential effects on retinal function, and increase excretion of calcium that can lead to possible osteoporosis and nephrolitiasis. The same caveats apply as for the high-protein, low-carbohydrate diet detailed in Chapter 4.

As mentioned above, there is also a specific problem with possible copper build-up on the SCD which would need to be carefully monitored, particularly in someone with an ASD. It has been reported that elevated serum copper levels can be linked to aggressive behaviour, particularly in the context of low plasma levels of zinc (Walsh *et al.* 1997).

Resources

A useful resource for those considering starting to use the SCD is the Elaine Gottschall website: www.breakingtheviciouscycle.info/index.htm. Her books, *Food and the Gut Reaction* (1987) and *Breaking the Vicious Cycle* (1994) are probably the best-known work on the SCD. Her website provides some information on the rationale and on how to implement the diet.

A number of cookbooks are also now available to help with cooking on the SCD (Conrad 2006; Prasad 2008), and there is a helpful website devoted to SCD cooking: www.scdrecipe.com.

There is also an autism-specific site: www.gottschallcenter.com, run by the Gottschall Autism Center, that has links to a number of video presentations concerning using the SCD in ASD.

Other useful sites are:

www.pecanbread.com

www.scdiet.org.

In the UK, a website www.scduk.co.uk provides information on a range of issues, recipes, and contact details on suppliers for SCD products in the UK.

Material on the SCD can be found on the Celiac.com website: www.celiac.com.

A recent article on using the SCD with autism ('Free the butterflies – the Specific Carbohydrate Diet and autism', by Carol Frilegh, published on 26 December 2007) can be accessed at: www.celiac.com/articles/21510/1/Free-the-Butterflies---The-Specific-Carbohydrate-Diet-and-Autism/Page1.html.

CHAPTER 7

The CF-GF Diet

Research on casein-free gluten-free diets was recommended as a priority area in the 2001 MRC research review (MRC 2001). Systematic study on CF-GF diets has yet to be funded at the time of writing – some seven years later. A proposal for the CANDAA (CAN Diet Affect Autism) study is awaiting funds. This is a project that has been proposed by the Nuffield Centre, University of Newcastle (see: www.research autism.net/pages/research/current_research). It has the approval and support of Research Autism, the new research of the UK National Autistic Society: www.researchautism.net/pages/welcome/home.ikml. At the time of writing, there is still an urgent need for proper evaluative research (see Millward *et al.* 2008).

A number of anecdotal accounts have been published with huge improvements reported in individual cases (see, for example, McCarthy 2007; Seroussi 1999). There is a considerable amount of material available describing this approach and its theoretical underpinnings from sources such as the ARU (University of Sunderland Autism Research Unit: http://osiris.sunderland.ac.uk/autism) and ANDI (Autism Network for Dietary Intervention: www.autismndi.com) websites.

What is it?

Although casein and gluten are different compounds and metabolic problems with either could arise, dietary interventions that have been used with ASD have typically involved the exclusion or limitation of both casein and gluten.

What is casein?

Casein is a protein found in milk. The word comes from the Latin for cheese: *caseus*. The molecular structure of casein is very similar to that of gluten. Both can be metabolized to produce opioid-like compounds called respectively caseomorphins and gluteomorphins. Some types of milk are thought to be potentially less likely to cause problems due to differences in the molecular structure of their casein, particularly 'A2' milk that has an amino acid substitution in the β-casein gene. Cowsmilk contains seven proteins that are of potential significance (α-, β- and K-casein, α- and β-lactoglobulin, lactoferrin and transferrin). A2 milk does not seem to result in any lowered allergic response (see Smith *et al.* 2004). Although there has been much media interest, the level of evidence supporting the likely benefits from A2 milk is currently quite weak (see Swinburn 2004).

Both transferrin and lactoferrin are important in binding iron from the bloodstream. Excess iron is a factor which helps bacteria to proliferate, so reduced levels of these proteins can lead to bacterial overgrowth. Transferrin levels have been found to be low in ASD (Chauhan *et al.* 2004). Lactoferrin, known as colostrum, has been produced from cowsmilk and is available as a commercial supplement product from various companies. Note that normal cowsmilk has little lactoferrin as milking cattle do not produce significant amounts once they have stopped suckling. Some conditions which result in iron build-up are more prevalent in Scandinavian and other Northern European countries (e.g. haemochromatosis or the 'Celtic curse': Raszeja-Wyszomirska *et al.* 2008).

Further research is required to examine whether there is a link between factors such as milk-free diet, transferrin levels, iron metabolism and ASD. It is possible that there was a difference in milk intake between the autistic and non-autistic children in the Chauhan *et al.* 2004 study – 5/19 autistic and 0/19 controls were gluten free so there were some explicit dietary differences, but no mention is made of milk exclusion or intake.

What is gluten?

Gluten is a protein that is found at high levels in a number of grains, particularly in wheat, barley and rye. It is thus found in most types of cereals, many types of bread, cakes and biscuits. Not all grains contain gluten. It is easy, however, for gluten contamination to arise where various grains are processed in the same mill. There are some specialist flourmills that only produce gluten-free products (see www.bobs-redmill.com).

There continues to be debate over the clinical role of gluten-free carbohydrates; however, grains such as oats are often well tolerated in a gluten-free diet (Peräaho *et al.* 2004a, 2004b). Examples of grains that do not contain gluten are amaranth, buckwheat, corn, millet, oats, quinoa, soybeans, sunflower seeds and tef (tef is an East African grain crop now also being cultivated in parts of the USA) (see Spaenij-Dekking, Kooy-Winkelaar and Koning 2005). Different types of grain have different levels of gluten and have different likelihoods of triggering gluten sensitivity reactions (for comparisons, see Vader *et al.* 2003). The way in which celiac disease patients react to grain is through lack of T cell tolerance to gluten, and the production of tissue transglutaminase. The reaction is dependent on the spacing between glutamine and proline in gluten from wheat, and to the similar amino acid pattern seen in the hordeins from barley and the secalins in rye. The lack of such a pattern in the avenins found in oats is probably the factor that accounts for the lesser chance of a celiac reaction being elicited (Vader *et al.* 2002).

What does a CF-GF diet claim to do?

There are various theories concerning possible problems with the presence of casein and gluten in the diet.

1. The 'leaky gut' theory: This has been proposed by various people – most notably by the research group working at the University of Sunderland headed by Paul Shattock (see

http://osiris.sunderland.ac.uk/autism) and the research group at the University of Oslo headed by Kalle Reichelt. For both of these groups, the principal problem is thought to be the passage of opioid-like compounds into the bloodstream across the lining of the intestine (Anderson *et al.* 2002; Reichelt and Knivsberg 2003). The development of interest in casein and gluten derived neuropeptides has been reviewed comprehensively elsewhere (Klavdieva 1996).

In Florida, at the University of Gainesville, Robert Cade (who funded his researches from the profits made on the invention of 'Gatorade') and colleagues have demonstrated the rapid uptake in the rat brain of β-casomorphin-7 injected into the bloodstream (Sun *et al.* 1999). This group have also conducted open trials which have shown considerable beneficial effects of milk exclusion in ASD (Cade *et al.* 2000).

If the opioid excess, leaky gut theory has validity, it should be useful to establish whether a particular child is excreting excess urinary opioids. We know from the animal work of Cade and others that circulating opioids in the bloodstream rapidly cross the blood–brain barrier and affect brain function. If excess opioids can be detected in urine, they would have been filtered out from the bloodstream by the kidneys and therefore there would be excessive circulating levels of exogenous opioids in the body.

2. The immune theory: In some conditions associated with ASD, including Down syndrome (Bonamico *et al.* 2001; Shamaly *et al.* 2007) and Williams syndrome (Giannotti *et al.* 2001), there is a high prevalence of celiac disease. Here, the affected person has antibodies that react to gluten – antiendomesial and antigliadin antibodies. The response to ingestion of gluten in such individuals is a true allergic response rather than a reaction to incomplete digestion coupled with increased intestinal permeability. Celiac seems an unlikely factor in most cases of ASD as the two studies which have examined levels of celiac antibodies in randomized ASD populations have not found celiac antibodies to be overrepresented (Black, Kaye and Jick 2002; Vazirian *et al.* 2007).

3. It is possible that the mechanism underpinning improvement is different from the rationale proposed for the diet – if, for example, the benefit was due to a reduction in lactose intake, removing milk products may prove beneficial, but the benefits of dietary restriction would be unrelated to a difficulty with casein or gluten digestion and could respond to a lactase supplement with equal benefit.

A recent study has suggested a possible association between L-2-Hydroxyglutaric aciduria and ASD (Zafeiriou *et al.* 2007). This inborn error of metabolism results from a difficulty in metabolizing certain sugars including galactose, a sugar uniquely derived from lactose found only in milk in the Western diet. It seems likely that for some cases at least, where removal of milk products has proven beneficial, the difference results from removal of lactose rather than from removal of casein.

One of the genes involved in L-2-Hydroxyglutaric aciduria, 3q26.1-q26.3, has the highest level of association with ASD so far reported with a two point LOD score of 4.31 (Auranen *et al.* 2002). If robust and replicable, this suggests that there is a subgroup of ASD in which inability to metabolize milk sugars is a treatable component of their disorder which may account for some cases who respond to the CF-GF diet.

Is this the same mechanism that causes celiac disease?

Celiac (also known as 'coeliac') disease is a condition where antibodies are produced by the immune system, which react specifically to gluten – these are called anti-endomesial and anti-gliadin antibodies (see Holtmeier and Caspary 2006). There is a simple blood test that can be requested by a paediatrician or general practitioner to detect the presence of these antibodies. Although there are cases of celiac disease in association with ASD, these are no more frequent than in the general population and not common enough to suggest that the primary mechanism by which such cases improve is due to gluten exclusion and removal of such an immune provocation (except in the case of the Down syndrome and Williams syndrome situations mentioned above).

Testing for celiac disease should be part of the assessment carried out in screening for potential dietary influences, but seems unlikely to be a significant factor in the majority of ASD cases. The apparent additive effects of casein and gluten exclusion also suggest that there is something different going on in these cumulative cases at least.

What is the evidence for CF-GF diets in ASD?

The Cochrane review of CF-GF dietary interventions in ASD found only two small adequate RCT trials of such interventions (Millward *et al.* 2008), and a further systematic review drew similar conclusions (Christison and Ivany 2006). Both recommended the need for good prospective larger-scale double-blinded studies. The methodology for such an approach has been tested in preliminary research (Elder *et al.* 2006).

A review of the seven published studies which were published up to 2000 found that the results were uniformly supportive of benefits from a CF-GF diet; however, all of the studies to that point had major methodological weaknesses (Knivsberg, Reichelt and Nodland 2000).

The only published study to date with reasonable rigour is a single-blinded randomized crossover study with objective rating of behaviour carried out over one year with ten autistic children who had been established to have high levels of urinary opioid excretion. This study found significant improvements in blind-rated assessments of autistic traits, non-verbal cognitive level (IQ), motor functioning, and on a range of parental report measures (Knivsberg *et al.* 2002).

Does it work?

There is no systematic research using a randomized controlled double-blind approach which has studied the casein-free, gluten-free, or CF-GF diet for ASD. This is the 'gold standard' level of research required in evidence-based medicine to establish proof of benefit.

Parent reports to the Autism Research Institute (ARI) on their standardized rating scale for effects of biomedical interventions gave the ratings shown in Table 7.1 from those who responded concerning these approaches.

Table 7.1 ARI casein- and gluten-free diet outcomes

	Worse	No change	Better	Number
Gluten-free and casein-free diet	3%	32%	65%	1446
Casein-free diet	2%	49%	49%	5574
Wheat-free diet	2%	50%	48%	3159

Are there potential problems with adopting a CF-GF diet?

One important recent finding is that in boys aged four to eight years who are on casein-free diets without adequate compensatory calcium intake, bone thickness as estimated by wrist x-ray is significantly less when compared to boys on minimally restricted or unrestricted diets (Hediger *et al.* 2007). This is obviously cross-sectional information on two populations, not a controlled study; however, it should urge caution in removing milk without ensuring adequate alternative sources of calcium.

As osteoporosis and kidney stone formation due to excessive calcium excretion are known problems with high-protein, low-carbohydrate diets and the CF-GF diet lowers carbohydrate with a probable compensatory increase in protein intake, similar precautions should be adopted to those recommended for a high-protein, low-carbohydrate diet in Chapter 4 and for the SCD (Chapter 6).

As for several of the other approaches discussed, it would also be sensible to limit oxalate intake on a CF-GF diet to minimize the possible risk of effects on bone growth and kidney function.

Much has been written in autism literature about possible problems with casein breakdown, and this has led to the use of milk exclusion being advocated and implemented as a dietary intervention. One problem which can arise through the exclusion of milk from the diet results from the removal of lactose, and consequent reduction in galactose.

Lactose is the disaccharide sugar found in milk, and galactose is a monosaccharide sugar that is produced from the metabolism of lactose. Glycolipids, which are important in brain development, typically contain galactose. There are a small number of rare genetic types of galactosemia (see Novelli and Reichardt 2000). In galactosemia there is a build-up of galactose in the body due to the absence of one of the three enzymes involved in its metabolism – galactose-1-phosphate uridyltransferase (GALT) being the most commonly reported defect.

As galactose is an important factor in the functioning of sulfation pathways, a functional deficiency due to milk exclusion can interfere with metabolic processes, and particularly with phenol degradation. As many of the foods which constitute the diet of someone who has adopted a low-carbohydrate lifestyle are high in phenols, and there is no other dietary source of galactose, specific lactose or galactose supplemention may be required by those with ASD who gain benefit from milk exclusion.

Could digestive enzymes be helpful?

A range of digestive enzyme products are available which help with the digestion of casein and gluten. A number of the more frequently used supplements are detailed in Table 7.2. Some have additional protein-digesting enzymes (known as proteases) that could increase opioid production in individuals who have changed to a ketogenic diet so should be used advisedly (assuming the opioid model has some merit).

Only EnZymAid provides a replacement for galactose. This would normally be provided by the breakdown of lactose but is depleted when on a dairy-free diet. Galactose supplementation should give additional benefits as galactose is involved in phenol degradation, unless the person in question has L-2-Hydroxyglutaric aciduria, a factor that should be considered given its overrepresentation in this population.

Digestive enzyme treatments are frequently recommended in the complementary literature (a general introduction can be found in Lee *et al*. 1998). There is a literature on their uses specifically with ASD (see, for example, Kidd 2002; McCandless 2007). There is evidence for anti-inflammatory effects of constituents in some of these products such as bromelain (Izaka *et al*. 1972) and papain. There are, to date, no controlled trials of digestive enzyme supplementation in the peer-reviewed clinical literature on ASD.

Karen DeFelice (2006, 2008) has been a strong advocate for the use of enzyme supplements with ASD, and has developed a useful website: www.enzymestuff.com/conditionpdd.htm.

Table 7.2 Digestive enzyme supplements

Product	Manufacturer	Contents
GlutenEase	Enzymedica See: www.enzymedica.com	DPP IV Protease; Amylase and Glucoamylase
Glutenzyme Plus	Biocare See: www.biocare.co.uk	Cellulase, Lactobacillus brevis, Lactobacillus acidophilus, Gluten Protease and Amylase
Peptizyde	Houston	Peptidase, Protease, Papain (from papaya)
AFP Peptizyde	Houston See: www.houston-enzymes.com	Peptidase, Protease, 2nd Protease (differs from Peptizyde in using proteases derived from fungi rather than fruit – should be less likely to cause problems for people with phenol and salicylate sensitivities)

Product	Manufacturer	Contents
Peptidase Complete	Kirkman Pharmaceuticals	Peptidase, Bromelain (from pineapple) Protease 4.5, Papain (from sulfite-free papaya) and Protease 6.0
EzZymAid	Kirkman Pharmaceuticals See: www.kirkmanlabs.com/products	Caso-glutenase, Bromelain, Acid Fast Protease, Lactase, Phytase and Galactose

Resources

Organized groups

The Food Allergy Network
11781 Lee Jackson Hwy, Suite 160
Fairfax, VA 22033-3309
Tel: +1 800 929 4040

American Celiac Society
PO Box 23455
New Orleans, LA 70183-0455
Tel: +1 504 737 3293

The Autism Network for Dietary Intervention (ANDI)
PO Box 335
Pennington, NJ 08534-0335
Tel: +1 609 737 8985
Fax: +1 609 737 8453

Celiac Sprue Association/USA, Inc.
PO Box 31700
Omaha, NE 68131-0700
Tel: +1 402 558 0600
+1 877 CSA-4-CSA

Celiac Disease Foundation
13251 Ventura Blvd., Suite 1
Studio City, CA 91604-1838
Tel: +1 818 990 2354

Gluten Intolerance Group
15110 10th Avenue SW, Suite A
Seattle, WA 98166-1820
Tel: +1 206 246 6652

Useful books

Case, S. (2006) *Gluten-Free Diet: A Comprehensive Resource Guide.* Case Nutrition Consulting: Regina, Saskachewan.

Compart, P.J. and Laake, D. (2007) *The Kid-Friendly ADHD and Autism Cookbook (The Ultimate Guide to the Gluten-Free Casein-Free Diet – What It Is, Why It Works, How To Do It).* Fair Winds Publishing: Gloucester, Maryland.

Corn, D. (2006) *Living Gluten-Free For Dummies.* For Dummies (John Wiley and Sons): New York.

Lewis, L. (1999) *Special Diets for Special Kids: Understanding and Implementing Special Diets to Aid in the Treatment of Autism and Related Developmental Disorders.* Jessica Kingsley Publishers: London.

Triumph Dining (2007) *The Essential Gluten-Free Grocery Guide.* Arlington, Virginia.

Triumph Dining (2008) *The Essential Gluten-Free Restaurant Guide* (3rd edn). Arlington, Virginia. (see www.triumphdining.com)

Useful websites

www.celiac.com
www.autismndi.com
www.gfcfdiet.com
www.nutritionandmind.com
www.glutenfreediet.ca/index.php

GLUTEN-FREE PRODUCTS NORTH AMERICA

www.glutenfree.com
www.glutenfreemall.com
www.glutensolutions.com

GLUTEN-FREE PRODUCTS UK

www.glutenfree-foods.co.uk
www.gffdirect.co.uk

EATING OUT IN THE UK AND EUROPE

www.gluten-free-onthego.com

CHAPTER 8

The Low Oxalate Diet

Why do I need to know about oxalates?

Oxalates are found as crystals in plants where they concentrate light and boost photosynthesis. Oxalates are thus found in many foods and drinks. Oxalate levels have recently been shown to be highly elevated in some people with autism. There are various possible reasons for this, the most likely being eating high-oxalate foods, an abnormal pattern of gut bacteria (particularly lack of *Oxalobacter formigenes*), certain fungal infections, certain fairly uncommon genetic conditions, and, rarely, drinking ethylene glycol (typically in anti-freeze).

High oxalate levels increase the risk of forming kidney stones. Kidney stones typically form through calcium building up around a kernel of oxalate. Oxalate intake thus needs to be controlled in dietary approaches such as low-carbohydrate diets that increase risk by increasing calcium excretion, and thus increase the risk of kidney stone formation (nephrolithiasis).

What are oxalates?

Oxalates are salts formed by the displacement of a hydrogen atom from a molecule of oxalic acid by a metal. Oxalic acid is found in high amounts in a range of foodstuffs including spinach, chocolate, sorrel, rhubarb, asparagus and nuts. Sorrel, a traditional herb, has particularly high levels of both oxalic acid and phenols. The high concentration of oxalic acid in rhubarb leaves is the reason they are toxic and inedible.

High levels can also be found in rice with certain infections such as the fungal infection *Rhizoctonia solani.*

A toxic source not usually part of the food chain is from ethylene glycol, found principally in anti-freeze, but also in inks and brake fluids. Drinking these can rapidly result in renal failure and CNS damage due to build-up of oxalic acid and calcium oxalate. This is occasionally a problem in young children where they have had access to such products, as these tend to be sweet tasting and can be mistaken for drinks. In the mid-1980s, there was a problem with certain wines having small amounts of ethylene glycol added to improve the taste (see: http://en.wikipedia.org/wiki/Diethylene_glycol).

Many of the problems associated with oxalate metabolism have been systematically reviewed (Williams and Smith 1968; Williams and Wilson 1990). Problems with oxaluria have been recognized for many years, being well described in British troops training in India in the Second World War, where kidney stones were commonly found to result from restricted fluid intake when coupled with higher than normal levels of consumption of high oxalate foods such as rhubarb, asparagus and chocolate which were in short supply in the UK (see Black 1945).

What is hyperoxaluria?

The definition simply means having excess amounts of oxalate/oxalic acid in urine. This can result from a variety of factors:

1. A number of dietary factors can be important including reduced fluid intake and ingestion of high oxalate foods.

2. Certain types of fungi can produce oxalates, in particular a number of types of fungi of the genus *Aspergillus.*

3. There are a number of genetic causes of hyperoxaluria, the two most common being the following:

   ○ Primary hyperoxaluria type 1. This is caused by alanine-glyoxylate aminotransferase deficiency/serine:pyruvate aminotransferase deficiency (mapped to 2q36-q37). Some cases respond to treatment with high-dose vitamin B6 (Will and Bijvoet 1979).

o Primary hyperoxaluria Type 2. This is caused by a defect in the glyoxylate reductase/hydroxypyruvate reductase gene (mapped to 9q12) characterized by excretion of L-glycerate (see De Pauw and Toussaint 1996; Kemper, Conrad and Muller-Wiefel 1997).

4. Lack of or deficient levels of oxalate binding bacteria such as *Oxalobacter formigenes.*

5. Ethelene glycol, most commonly used as anti-freeze in cars, is converted to oxalic acid by the body. There have been poisonings due to deliberate drinking of anti-freeze, but also through adulteration of white wine with ethylene glycol to improve the taste. This suggests that there may be some positive gustatory effects of oxalates.

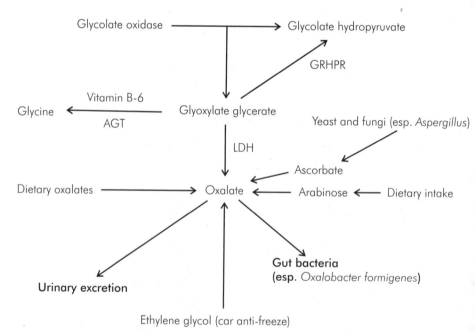

GRHPR: Glyoxylate reductase hydroxypyruvic reductase; AGT: Alanine glyoxylate aminotransferase; LDH: Lactate dehydrogenase

Figure 8.1 Oxalate metabolism

How is oxalate metabolized?

Figure 8.1 is a flow chart of oxalate metabolism. A variety of factors affect oxalate levels in the body including intake of high-oxalate foods, the presence of oxalate-binding bacteria in the GI tract (affected by antibiotic usage), presence of oxalate-forming fungi, fluid intake, and levels of vitamin B6.

Can oxalate levels be tested?

The simple answer to this is yes. A number of laboratories provide testing of oxalic acid levels in urine that is an indicator of body oxalate levels. Evidence to date suggests that oxalate levels in many autistics are significantly elevated. The Great Plains Laboratory (www.greatplains-laboratory.com) cite a mean oxalate level in a tested autistic population (N=100) which is some five times normal control values (N=16), but with wide variation in individual levels (90.1+/−75.7 vs 15.7+/−10.8 mmol/mol creatinine).

What do oxalates do?

Oxalates are only found at low levels in animal tissue and are exclusively of plant origin. In plants, the crystals are involved in concentrating light for photosynthesis. It may also be that oxalates evolved as a protective mechanism in some plants against being consumed by animals. There do not appear to be any major positive physiological effects of oxalates in the human body. They do act as minor chelators for aluminium, mercury and lead, and regulate the levels of calcium in the endoplasmic reticulum so could also be involved in the regulation of peroxisome formation; however, they do not appear to play a central role in any of these processes.

Most studies to date have investigated the negative effects of oxalate excess. High levels impair citric acid cycle function through interference with pyruvate carboxylase, and can also impair ATP production through glycolysis, thus reducing energy for muscle function.

Oxalate build-up is involved in various aspects of bodily function, but is particularly relevant to the formation of kidney stones and results in an increased likelihood of obesity (Lemann *et al.* 1996; Taylor, Stampfer and Curhan 2005).

Low oxalate diets have been advocated for a number of years, particularly for people who are at risk of forming kidney stones, and for those with vulval pain. To lower their chances of kidney stone formation, people at risk are advised to limit oxalate intake from foods to 40–50 mg per day, and to avoid a high intake of oxalate precursors such as vitamin C (being encouraged to limit intake to less than 2 g per day). Higher levels of vitamin C ingestion result in higher levels of oxalate excretion (see Levine *et al.* 1996).

The link between oxalate levels and risk of kidney stone formation (nephrolithiasis) is inferred from various studies that show a correlation between obesity, oxalate levels and increased risk of stone formation (see Curhan 1999). Interestingly, increasing intake of vitamin B6 lowers oxalate levels (Curhan *et al.* 1999; Menon and Mahle 1982). Oxalate levels are more strongly associated with likelihood of kidney stone formation than calcium levels (Massey and Smith 1993).

Mineral levels are important for oxalate clearance. In particular, calcium and magnesium supplementation has been shown to have major beneficial effects on oxalate clearance after loading with oxalate-rich foods (Liebman and Costa 2000).

From the above, it would seem sensible if embarking on a low oxalate diet to supplement with calcium, magnesium and vitamin B6, and to keep to a low intake of vitamin C.

The low oxalate diet in ASD – what does it aim to do?

Biochemically, excess oxalate impairs the body's ability to break down protein by impairing the pyruvate kinase step in glycolysis. If this mechanism is not working properly in someone who has adopted a low-carbohydrate diet, they may run into problems due to lack of glycogen. This is often a transient effect of a low-carbohydrate diet in someone without a problem with oxalates who will experience, as discussed above, faster onset of fatigue during exercise (Greenhaff *et al.* 1987a, 1987b, 1988).

The following is a list of factors that could suggest oxalate issues in an ASD child. This list has been drawn up based on parents' reports of benefits observed on a low oxalate diet in the Autism Oxalate Project detailed below.

How common any such improvements may prove to be is not known at this time.

Reported changes in physiological factors: Improvement in urinary problems including urinary urgency and frequency, genital pain, over-extended bladder and formation of kidney stones – as there is a robust literature on low oxalate diet reducing vulval pain, this finding is consistent with the literature, reduction in outbursts of bad behaviour or of pain within minutes to within a couple of hours of eating, improvement in constipation or diarrhoea unresponsive to other therapy, improvement in physical growth (even that which is responsive to growth hormone therapy) and reduced abdominal bloating unresponsive to other treatment or diet.

Reported changes in behaviours: Improvements in expressive speech and reduced obsessive behaviour.

Reported changes linked to supplements: Changes in function or behaviour that follow use of Miralax or Glycolax, reduced problems with glycine (DMG, TMG), reduced intolerance to sulfur supplements, craving high oxalate foods, biotin issues (but maybe not responsive to biotin or even behaviour that gets worse on biotin) and possibly odd reactions to calcium like self-stimulatory or other repetitive behaviour.

Reported problems on the diet: New problems developing whenever nuts, legumes or soy are introduced and, in one case, possible seizure.

What is the evidence?

At present, a number of families in the USA are taking part in a study of the usefulness of low oxalate diets in ASD – the Autism Oxalate Project which is being coordinated by Susan Owens from the Stillpoint Integrative Medicine Center, and the Husson Science Research Institute in Temecula, California (see: www.stillpointhealth.com/LowOxalate Diet-HelpandSuggestion.html). To date, the evidence comes from participants in this project and Owens' presentations. These are a 'work in progress', and no peer-reviewed publications have as yet appeared. As can be seen by looking through the list of reported benefits, many of these are improvements in bowel and bladder problems as would be expected and differences in response to calcium intake. Most of the others are improvements in the child's ability to tolerate foods to which they had previously shown sensitivities or in their response to other CAM supplements.

One particular anaerobic bacterium, *Oxalobacter formigenes*, absorbs oxalates, helping to prevent hyperoxaluria. This bacterium is, unfortunately, inactivated by many common antibiotics (Duncan *et al.* 2002). In cystic fibrosis where there is aggressive pharmacotherapy of the condition, *Oxalobacter* cannot usually be cultured (Sidhu *et al.* 1998). As many children with ASD have received multiple courses of antibiotics, there may be impairment in their ability to control oxalate levels through this mechanism.

There are developments in terms of possible pharmacological methods of binding oxalates and improving excretion. One company in particular, OxThera Inc. (see www.oxthera.com) is developing two products: Oxabact, a supplement of live *Oxalobacter formigenes*, the bacterium which lowers oxalate levels in both plasma and urine; and Oxazyme, an oxalate-degrading enzyme. At the present time neither product has been trialled for use in hyperoxaluric ASD. From animal studies, *Oxalobacter formigenes* has the ability to reverse hyperoxaluria rapidly (Sidhu *et al.* 2001).

A number of gut bacteria other than *Oxalobacter* degrade oxalates, including *lactobacillus acidophilus* and *bifidobacterium lactis* (Azcarate-Peril *et al.* 2006), so an appropriately targeted general probiotic supplementation programme (see Young and Huffman 2003) may be useful in reducing oxalate levels. In general, reduction of normal gut bacteria resulting from repeated antibiotic use is likely to impair the body's ability to process and excrete oxalates.

Resources

The Oxalosis and Hyperoxaluria Foundation
201 East 19th Street, Suite 12E
Tel: +1 212 777 0470
Fax: +1 212 777 0471
Toll Free: +1 800 OHF 8699
Website: www.ohf.org/index.html
Email: kimh@ohf.org

The foundation website has excellent downloadable lists of foodstuffs by oxalate level (updated 2008).

A useful background document on the low oxalate diet in autism can be found at: www.stillpointhealth.com/LowOxalateDiet-HelpandSuggestion.html.

Further information is on the Low Oxalate Diet website: http://lowoxalate.info/index.html.

A more general introduction to oxalates can be found at: www.vulvarpainfoundation.org/vpfoxalate.htm.

The Vulvar Pain Foundation also produce *The Low Oxalate Cookbook – Two* which can be obtained from their website.

An introduction to the low oxalate diet and how to dovetail this with other restriction diet approaches can be found at: Trying_Low_Oxalates@yahoo-groups.com.

Ixion Biotechnology is a Florida-based company that specializes in developing treatments for metabolic disorders with particular emphases on oxalate control and stem-cell control of diabetes: www.ixion-biotech.com.

CHAPTER 9

The Low Glutamate Diet/GARD (Glutamate-Aspartate Restricted Diet)

What is it?

Glutamate is a non-essential amino acid. This means that there are no obvious effects of not consuming it as a part of the diet. It can be made in the body through the digestion of glutamate-containing proteins; it is also an excitatory neurotransmitter which is found everywhere in the central nervous system (CNS).

A low glutamate or glutamate-aspartate restricted diet is one that restricts intake of glutamate and similar molecular compounds such as aspartate. A large amount has been written about possible problems resulting from MSG (monosodium glutamate) as an excitotoxin (see, for example, Blaylock 1997). A number of clinicians have suggested glutamate restriction as a dietary approach to the management of autism. The relationship between dietary intake of glutamate and CNS levels is not a strong one under normal circumstances as, typically, only limited amounts of glutamate cross the blood–brain barrier and enter the nervous system (Smith 2000).

If there was a difference in membrane permeability that results from an abnormality of polyunsaturated fatty acid levels, for example, as has been suggested in ASD, the effects might be different. There is good evidence for changes in metabolic rate due to differences in CNS temperature having effects on glutamate perfusion across the blood–brain barrier (see Gisolfi and Mora 2000). As there appears to be a high prevalence of oxidative phosphorylation defects in ASD and one of the roles of oxidative phosphorylation is to alter temperature, this could be an important factor in glutamate perfusion in ASD (James *et al.* 2004).

A range of other factors such as genetic defects in aquaporin-4 (Zhou *et al.* 2008) can affect blood–brain barrier development and function and could increase the impact of peripheral glutamate levels on brain glutamate. Viral exposure at certain critical points in early brain development can also affect the functioning of aquaporin-4 (Fatemi *et al.* 2008a, 2008b). As aquaporin-4 is involved in glial cell migration, neural signal transduction and brain oedema (Verkman *et al.* 2006), it may have a major effect in neural development. To date this has not been linked to abnormalities of glutamatergic function. Our understanding of aquaporins and their functions is very recent. Peter Agre of Johns Hopkins University in Baltimore shared the Nobel Prize for chemistry in 2003 for the discovery and investigation of aquaporin channels (Agre 2006). Defects in aquaporin-4 are known to occur in some of the neuromuscular conditions that have been associated with ASD and in epilepsy (Benga 2006; Obeid and Herrmann 2006).

A number of genetic conditions associated with ASD affect the development of CNS glutamate receptors, the best known being Fragile-X syndrome, a 'triplet repeat expansion' condition in which there has been overreplication of a small fragment of the X-chromosome resulting in inactivation of several gene products (Goodlin-Jones *et al.* 2004). In Fragile-X, one consequence is a failure of development of the metabotropic mGluR5 receptor, one type of glutamate receptor found widely in the central nervous system. It would appear that the main functional effect of the gene expansion is to interfere with metabotropic glutamate receptor-coupled pathways involving mGluR5 (Bear 2005).

There has been a significant leap forward in our recent understanding of metabotropic glutamate receptor function (Ferraguti and Shigemoto 2006), and in how these differences affect early brain development (Antar *et al.* 2004).

Various abnormalities of glutamate have been reported in autism. Increased numbers of AMPA (amino-3-hydroxy-5-methyl-4-isoxazole propionic acid) receptors have been identified at autopsy (Purcell *et al.*

2001). Differences have also been found in a number of genes which are involved in glutamatergic function (Jamain *et al.* 2002; Ramoz *et al.* 2004).

What does the diet claim to do?

A low glutamate diet aims to reduce dietary intake of both free and bound glutamate. Typically it also tries to limit aspartame intake – an artificial sweetener with a similar biochemical structure, and putative mode of action. Some genes involved in glutamate transport are also known to be involved in aspartate transport.

Glutamate is ubiquitous in the human body and is a neurotransmitter found throughout the nervous system, unlike the better studied neurotransmitter systems that employ serotonin and dopamine.

What is the evidence?

There is limited evidence concerning the possible role of reducing dietary glutamate in ASD. A number of conditions that result in ASD are known to involve abnormalities of glutamate metabolism in the brain. Best known is the absence of the mGluR5 receptor in Fragile-X syndrome (Bear, Huber and Warren 2004). Two studies have also found abnormalities in the genes for the mGluR6 receptor (see Freitag 2006).

The uses of mGluR5 blocking agents in animal models of Fragile-X syndrome have provided strong theoretical and empirical support (Bear *et al.* 2004). Results are showing remarkable reversal of symptomology with apparent improvement in learning, memory and social behaviour (see Dölen *et al.* 2007).

There is also the link between autism and the aspartate-glutamate carrier SLC25A12 gene that is involved in mitochondrial function (Segurado *et al.* 2005). Oxidative stress in mitochondria and abnormalities of mitochondrial glutamate are reported in various neurodegenerative conditions, and this seems a promising line of future research (Trushina and McMurray 2007). Several studies now demonstrate oxidative phosphorylation differences in ASD associated with mitochondrial defects (Oliveira *et al.* 2005; Poling *et al.* 2006; Rossignol and Bradstreet 2008; Shoffner, Hyams and Langley 2008). Oxidative phosphorylation is the process that generates heat to maintain body temperature and adenosine triphosphate for energy (Wallace 2005).

Build-up of lactic acid and an abnormal lactate/pyruvate ratio are metabolic indications of abnormal mitochondrial function. These have both been reported in a significant proportion of ASD cases in one large series (Correia *et al.* 2006).

An epidemiological study of ASD prevalence across Portugal has reported mitochondrial respiratory chain disorders in a surprisingly high proportion of cases (20 per cent) (Oliviera *et al.* 2007).

It appears that mitochondrial dysfunction can both result in oxidative stress, as suggested above, or result from it – in mouse models, at least, mitochondrial dysfunction can be produced by induction of insulin resistance through modifying the diet (Bonnard *et al.* 2008). The recent interest has been in cases where mitochondrial dysfunction may be part of a causal chain resulting in ASD. The basis being proposed is that mitochondrial defects predispose the individual to risk from other exposures. Further work is required to clarify the mechanisms here as some of the work to date suggests that the metabolic disturbances may in some cases be a consequence rather than a cause.

Resources

DogtorJ.com
http://dogtorj.tripod.com/id107.html

The United Mitochondrial Disease Foundation
8085 Saltsburg Road, Suite 201
Pittsburgh, PA 15239
Tel: +1 412 793 8077
US toll free: +1 888 317 UMDF (8633)
Fax: +1 412 793 6477
Email: info@umdf.org
Website: www.umdf.org/site/c.dnJEKLNqFoG/b.3041929

CHAPTER 10

The Low Phenylalanine Diet

What is it?

Phenylalanine is an amino acid found in nature and at high levels in certain foodstuffs. The low phenylalanine diet is designed to allow people with an inherited recessive metabolic defect of phenylalanine metabolism (known as phenylketonurea or PKU) to cope with a diet that is naturally low in this amino acid. PKU results from the lack of a liver enzyme, phenylalanine hydroxylase, which in normal circumstances converts phenylalanine to tyrosine. Without dietary restriction, there is a build-up of phenylpyruvic acid. PKU affects around 1 in 10,000 liveborn infants. Before the introduction of dietary treatment for PKU, it was a common cause of both learning disability and ASD. More recently, with the use of the Guthrie test to detect PKU in infants shortly after birth, problems associated with having PKU have largely disappeared in Western countries.

A significant number of people have subclinical differences in their ability to metabolize phenylalanine, something called hyperphenylalaninaemia. At present, no systematic management or dietary advice is given to those who are hyperphenylalaninaemic and who have lesser deficits in phenylalanine metabolism. It is likely that limiting dietary intake may be beneficial to them, and particularly to their unborn children if they are girls.

The children of girls with this pattern are at risk of problems, particularly if their mothers have ingested high amounts of phenylalanine during pregnancy – hyperphenylalaninaemic women who are trying to conceive should seek dietary advice. One potential source of such exposure is from aspartame-based artificial sweeteners, many of which are 50 per cent phenylalanine. As aspartame and aspartame-like sweeteners are extensively used in the food industry and are common constituents of diet products, it is possible for significant levels of aspartame to be taken in the early stages of pregnancy that are likely to cause high levels of exposure to the unborn baby. In a baby who is not carrying the genes predisposing him/her to hyperphenylalaninaemia this is not problematic; however, where the child has the maternal genes predisposing to this problem, the effects will be more severe than in the mother, as levels of *in utero* exposure will be considerably higher.

What does it claim to do?

There is good evidence that dietary intervention from shortly after birth can markedly improve predicted outcome in those with PKU (for a recent overview, see de Baulny *et al.* 2007). There is no evidence on the beneficial effects of limiting phenylalanine intake in those who do not have full-blown PKU.

What is required?

Before considering this type of dietary intervention, it is important to have the person assessed to evaluate the nature and extent of any difficulty in metabolizing phenylalanine. A larger number of independent gene differences are sufficient to cause PKU (for a review see Aitken 2008). As a recessive disorder, the prevalence of the genes that express as PKU is high – around 1 in 50 of the general population carries a PKU allele, with approximately 1 in 25,000 liveborn children being affected.

A diet that is rich in vitamins, minerals and other essential nutrients but low in phenylalanine is needed. Phenylalanine is found at high levels in animal proteins so it is important to limit intake of beef, pork, chicken, fish, eggs, cheese and milk. There are also significant levels in most nuts and nut butters. High levels of phenylalanine are found in a number of artificial sweeteners – those based on aspartame.

A good, low phenylalanine diet usually requires proprietary supplementation, but centres on fresh fruit and vegetables (but with limited amounts of corn, peas, rice, potatoes, regular pasta and bread).

It is important to seek dietetic advice if embarking on a low phenylalanine diet. The complexities of the diet are such that this type of diet should be supervised by a competent dietician and would only be indicated where there was clear evidence of an inborn error of phenylalanine metabolism.

What is the evidence?

Interestingly, the evidence concerning the low phenylalanine diet for PKU is less strong than would be the case were the link to be discovered today. Few studies with good designs have been carried out (see Poustie *et al.* 1999). This is because studies comparing no diet with dietary intervention are now unethical given our level of understanding about the condition. The prediction concerning the effects of a randomized trial would be a negative effect for the no-diet group. The evidence from prospective non-randomized studies provides convincing evidence of the beneficial effects for those with PKU, and, as mentioned earlier, there is evidence that failure to detect PKU and not instituting a diet can result in developmental delay and ASD (Vanli *et al.* 2006).

To date no studies have been carried out on the effects of restricting phenylalanine intake on those with lesser defects in phenylalanine metabolism, on outcome of improved dietary control for subclinical cases during pregnancy, or on whether such individuals are disproportionately represented in the mothers of those with ASD.

One study (Aldred *et al.* 2003) has shown significantly elevated levels of several amino acids in ASD – glutamic acid, phenylalanine, asparagine, tyrosine, alanine, and lysine. The authors concluded that the findings indicated a familial disorder of amino acid metabolism.

A low phenylalanine diet is also typically low in long-chain polyunsaturated fatty acids (LCPUFAs) such as arachidonic acid (AA) (omega-6) and docosahexaenoic acid (DHA) (omega-3). LCPUFAs are essential for the formation of cell membranes and myelination of the brain and peripheral nervous system. One study of 12-month supplementation with LCPUFAs in PKU found enhanced levels of docosahexaenoic acid (DHA), an increase in lipid levels in blood cell membranes and enhanced visual function on electrophysiological assessment (Agostoni *et al.* 2000). A further study by the same group, published in 2003 (Agostoni *et al.* 2003), found that group differences seen in the first study had disappeared three years after ceasing supplementation, suggesting the need for ongoing supplementation if benefits are to be maintained.

Carnitine

Another factor that is deficient unless specifically supplemented in those on a PKU diet is carnitine. The production of carnitine requires precursors that are derived from phenylalanine. Carnitine is produced from lysine, a dietary amino acid which, as we have seen (Aldred *et al.* 2003), is typically elevated in PKU; this combination of findings suggests that there is a specific problem in the conversion of lysine to carnitine.

Serum carnitine levels have been found to be lowered in ASD in general compared to normal controls (Filipek *et al.* 2004). This seems to be correctable by appropriate oral supplementation (Vilaseca *et al.* 1993). Levels are also low in Rett syndrome and also appear to respond to supplementation (Ellaway *et al.* 2001).

Lowered carnitine levels are seen in a number of different situations – as a consequence of sodium valproate use in the treatment of epilepsy (Verrotti *et al.* 1999), and in type 1 diabetes (Mamoulakis *et al.* 2004), both of which should be considered as possible factors if lowered levels are found. Levels are also low in Rett syndrome and also appear to respond to supplementation (Ellaway *et al.* 2001). It seems likely that the beneficial effects of supplementation are a consequence of the general protective effects which l-carnitine confers against the consequences of oxidative stress (Rajasekar and Anuradha 2007).

Are there developments in the management of difficulties with phenylalanine metabolism?

A number of developments are leading to improvements in the management of people with difficulties in metabolizing phenylalanine. Most relevant to possible dietary management are:

1. The development of more acceptable phenylalanine-free foods (see Macdonald *et al.* 2004) – low phenylalanine diets are historically quite unpalatable, so the development of better tasting alternatives helps to maintain people on their diets.

2. Improved cell membrane integrity through long-chain polyunsaturated fatty acid supplementation as an adjunct (Agostoni *et al.* 2000). This has been shown to be of additional benefit in stabilizing people on a low phenylalanine diet.

3. Reducing intestinal uptake of phenylalanine by the use of enzymes such as purified phenylalanine ammonia-lyase (Kim *et al.* 2004) also appears to be of value in reducing effects from phenylalanine ingestion.

Resources

Useful books

Schuett, V. (2003) *Low Protein Food List for PKU.* Hemlock Printers: Burnaby, Brishish Columbia.

Schuett, V. and Corry, D. (2005) *Apples to Zucchini: A Collection of Favorite Low Protein Recipes.* Delta Printing Solutions: Valencia, California.

Useful websites

In the UK, the NSPKU provides excellent dietary information that can be used by members, in conjunction with a dietician, and information on what is available on prescription. These can be downloaded from their website at: www.nspku.org/dietary_information.htm.

www.myspecialdiet.com is a site which both markets a wide range of foods for individuals who have specialized metabolic requirements such as phenylketonurea, maple syrup urine disease, homocystinuria, tyrosinemia, methylmalonic academia and celiac disease, and provides access to a variety of online articles and resources.

www.childrenshospital.org/newenglandconsortium/RMWebsite/PKU Guide/PKUGuide.htm is a particularly useful site for low phenylalanine recipes.

> The phenylalanine-free diet discussed here is very different from all of the other dietary interventions that we discuss and should only be undertaken where there is clear evidence of a problem in metabolizing phenylalanine, and good dietetic support to advise and help with the implementation of the diet.
>
> Unless there is an inborn metabolic defect, phenylalanine should not be excluded or restricted in the diet.

CHAPTER 11

The Low Phenol Diet

What is it?

A low phenol diet is one which restricts intake of highly phenolic foods. High levels of phenolic compounds are found in a range of foods and drinks, and a detailed listing should be consulted for dietary guidance (see, for example: www.zipworld.com.au/~ataraxy/Amines_list.html, or Seroussi 1999).

The foods which are high in phenols are difficult to classify into a simple group other than that they are largely fruits and vegetables – rhubarb, spinach, Brussels sprouts, beetroot, peanuts, cocoa, soya, blackberries, blueberries and wheat are all high natural sources. Sorrel, a traditional herb, has particularly high levels of phenols and oxalic acid.

What does it claim to do?

It is recognized that some individuals show reactions to phenols and natural salicylates in their diet. It has been demonstrated that an enzyme pathway, phenol sulfotransferase, which is involved in phase two liver detoxification, is primarily involved. This system appears to function abnormally in many ASD children. These children also excrete lower than normal levels of sulfate, sulfite and thiosulfite but increased levels of thiocyanate. This could indicate a higher body burden of cyanide as this is a rate-limiting factor in the production of thiocyanate (see Figure 11.1). As we have discussed, a number of other factors can increase cyanide levels, with passive smoking and cassava consumption being possible culprits.

Phenols are similar in structure to salicylates, which are found naturally in most citrus fruits and in many proprietary painkillers. Phenols are also found in large amounts in many processed foods in the form of preservatives (for example in the manufacture of wines and pastrami). Many of the synthetic phenols used as agricultural fertilizers also contain nitro/nitrite/nitrate groups.

Work by Rosemary Waring and colleagues at the University of Birmingham have examined sulfur metabolism (Alberti *et al.* 1999; Waring and Klovrza 2000), and, more specifically, the role of the enzyme known as phenolsulphotransferases (PSTs). PSTs are involved both in catecholamine function in the central nervous system, and in the metabolism of both phenols and salicylates. The function of PSTs as they are involved in phenol degradation can be affected by a number of dietary factors such as bioflavonoids (Ghazali and Waring 1999).

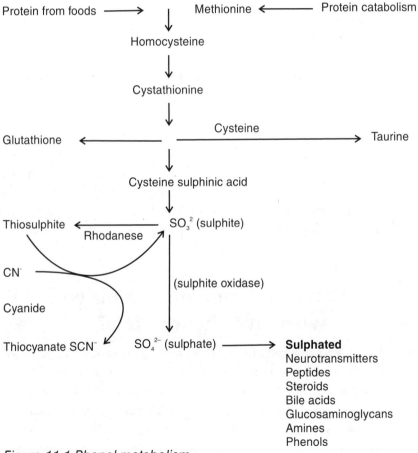

Figure 11.1 Phenol metabolism

What is the evidence?

As discussed, there is good evidence for differences in phenol metabolism in ASD (see, for example, Alberti *et al.* 1999; Waring and Klovrza 2000). These differences may be important in the production of oxidative damage to the ASD central nervous system (Evans *et al.* 2008). Degradation of phenolic compounds by sulfate conjugation is important in the metabolism of a range of phenolic compounds from foods and in addition in the metabolism of endogenous factors such as catecholamine neurotransmitters, steroids, bile acids, and of a number of phenolic and aromatic drugs and xenobiotics (see, for review, McFadden 1996). Many of these systems can be impaired when galactose is not present, and as the only dietary source of galactose is from lactose found in milk, problems with phenolic foods often arise from CF-GF diets.

Anecdotal reports of the benefits of using Epsom salts (magnesium sulphate) baths, or creams to improve sulphation pathways in ASD are common (see, for examples: www.bbbautism.com/epsom_condensed_plaintext.htm). To date, however, no systematic research has been published on this approach, or of benefits which may result from its use.

One point to be borne in mind is that the frequent use of Epsom salts baths is very drying to the skin and can result in skin becoming cracked or irritated. This can be avoided by the addition of olive oil to the bathwater and should be avoidable if creams are used instead.

Are there any potential problems with low phenol diets?

Phenols have been shown to be important in control of cholesterol levels in the blood (see Gimeno *et al.* 2002). Reducing phenol levels could increase cholesterol. A second potential interaction between phenol regulation and other factors in ASD management, based on bovine research at least, is that the active form of vitamin B6 (known as pyridoxal 5-phosphate or P5P) which is taken by many in high doses can have a negative effect on the functioning of the PST pathway (Bartzatt and Beckman 1994).

Resources

For a simple listing of phenol levels in different foodstuffs, see Karyn Seroussi's (1999) book *Unraveling the Mystery of Autism and Pervasive Developmental Disorder: A Mother's Story of Research and Recovery.*

A useful website dealing with salicylates and providing a useful food listing is: http://salicylatesensitivity.com.

A number of products are available which selectively bind and remove phenols from the body; three of the better-known are listed in Table 11.1.

Table 11.1 Phenol-lowering supplements

Product	Manufacturer	Contents
V-Gest	Enzymedica See: www.enzymedica.com	Amylase, Alpha-Galactosidase, Cellulase, Glucoamylase, Protease, Maltase, Invertase, Lactase, Lipase, Pectinase with Phytase, Hemicellulase and Xylanase
No-Phenol	Houston See: www.houstonni.com www.enzymestuff.com/ nofenolfile.htm	'Zyphenase', Xylanase and 'CereCalase' (hemicellulase, beta-glucanase, phytase)
Phenol Assist	Kirkman Pharmaceuticals See: www.kirkmanlabs.com/ products/enzymes/phe nol/phenol_bp835.html	Xylenase, 'CereCalase', Cellulase, BetaGlucanase, Phytase, Alpha-Amylase, Glucoamylase and Alpha-Galactosidase

CHAPTER 12

The Body Ecology Diet

What is it?

The Body Ecology Diet (BED) is a recent dietary approach to ASD, which was devised by US dietary 'guru' Donna Gates (see Gates 2006).

This is a recent dietary approach to working with ASD. There are no published studies or reports on its efficacy.

The BED approach draws on a number of specific dietary models, providing a synthesis of several approaches. The general approach is low dairy, low carbohydrate and low sugar so adheres to the basic principles that appear to underpin many of the more successful models. It does not appear to push ketosis, but focuses more on the concept of chronic problems such as ASD resulting from some form of GI overgrowth. Adherence to the general diet advised may lead to ketosis as maintaining protein and fat intake while reducing sugar and carbohydrate will encourage this process; however, the level of carbohydrate intake may still be too high.

The principal dietary models that the BED claims to be based on are the macrobiotic diet, the raw foods diet, the Weston A. Price diet, the D'Adamo 'Eat Right for Your Type' blood type diet, and the principles of food combining found in the Hay diet.

Various foods are recommended as being particularly beneficial such as coconut kefir – a high-carbohydrate probiotic drink cultured from the water extracted from young coconuts (this contains approximately 1 g of carbohydrate per 10 ml of kefir). There is a strong emphasis on consuming raw or minimally processed foods and unpasteurized 'raw' butter from grass-fed cattle which is high in conjugated linoleic acid.

What does it claim to do?

This diet combines a number of approaches that should be helpful, particularly to those individuals who are troubled by gut dysbiosis. Similar benefits should be seen to those from a number of the other approaches we have discussed. Claims for benefit are made in the literature produced by Body Ecology and a brochure specifically on its use with ASD can be downloaded from their website along with parent testimonials and a video presentation. Link from: http://body ecology.com/autism.php.

What is the evidence?

There is no evidence in the peer-reviewed published literature that gives support to this approach as being particularly likely to be of specific benefit in ASD.

It is not clear that this approach is likely to help with lipophilic toxin release, or provides any specific additional benefit other than the level of probiotic support that is often provided on other dietary regimes through the use of bacterial supplements to rebalance gut flora.

Resources

The Body Ecology website: www.bodyecologydiet.com.

A useful description of the Body Ecology Diet can be found through the ANDI website at: www.autismndi.com/news/display.asp?content=news& shownews=20040721140600.

This site also provides a link to a downloadable table of allowed and not allowed foods on the BED.

CHAPTER 13

The Rotation Diet

What is it?

There are various forms of rotation diet. The 'rotation diet' was originally developed as a weight-loss approach by Mark Katahn (Katahn 1987). It relied on the idea of rotating types of food and caloric intake from day to day to maintain interest in foods despite cutting calories, a second aim being to reduce the likelihood of an immune food reaction. In some respects this is similar to the earlier Hay food-combining diet developed in the 1920s by the New York physician Dr William Howard Hay (see Habgood 1997) which was popularized by the late British actor John Mills. The Hay approach was not primarily for weight control but said to improve general health.

On the Hay diet only certain combinations of foods can be consumed during the same meal. The principal rule is effectively separating carbohydrate and protein consumption. The rules are fairly simple but there is no clear nutritional rationale and some confusing prescriptions given the general rule – you can have meat, cheese and soyabean products together, while the last two may be high carbohydrate.

Basic rotation diet principles (Katahn)

On a four-day rotation diet, for example, no one food is eaten again until the fifth day. If a banana were eaten in the first day of the cycle, you would not be able to eat another until the fifth day.

Foods from the same food group may be eaten every second day – you could choose to eat a different cereal grain once every other day. So you could have wheat on day one, barley on day three, quinoa on day five and so on.

A specific food should only be eaten once in any given day. If you eat cornflakes for breakfast, no other corn-based foods – sweetcorn, creamed corn, tortillas, polenta, popcorn, etc. – should be eaten that day.

The first two principles are essential, even for those with a very limited selection of tolerated foods. The last principle is important for those who need to identify hidden food allergies, manage known food allergies, and prevent new food allergies from developing.

It is important to eliminate a known allergen completely for a minimum of 30 days before adding it into a rotation. Often tolerance for the foods can be regained (www.parentsofallergicchildren.org/principl.htm).

As used with ASD, rotational diets are more to do with improving immune function than changing food or caloric intake. Several basic principles apply:

1. Reduce intake of foods likely to contain toxic chemicals.

   Packaged foods, particularly in plastic wrapping, which have various potential contaminants, from phthalates to carbon tetracholoride, should where possible be replaced by fresh or frozen equivalents. Intake of processed foods and soft drinks should be minimized.

   Surface waxes, sprays and gas residues should be removed from fruit and vegetables before use with some form of non-toxic cleanser. Try to minimize use of refined sugar and flour products. Minimize use of margarine and increase intake of non-hydrogenated oils and butter.

2. Keep a balance of food groups in the diet, with a combination of adequate fibre, complex carbohydrates, proteins, and other essential minerals and vitamins from fresh fruits and vegetables.

3. Try to avoid using cookware likely to release potentially toxic materials into foods – aluminium, non-stick or cast-iron

cookware. Instead, try where possible to use stainless steel, glass or enamelled ceramic cookware.

4. Aim to avoid yeast and fungi where possible. Yeast and fungal spores are endemic – they can be found virtually anywhere, as most people discover when cleaning the inner recesses of the refrigerator, but tend to thrive best in moist warm places. Foods which tend to harbour spores – the surfaces of fruits and vegetables, seeds, pulses, rice and grains – should be washed before use. Dried foods – nuts, seeds, rice and dried beans – can be dry heated then stored in the freezer before use to minimize contamination.

5. Use of fermented foods (such as vinegars, cheeses, sausages such as salami and kabanos, pierogi, sauerkraut, kimchi, fish sauces, tofu, soy sauce and leavened breads) should be limited.

What does it claim to do?

The principal benefit of the rotation diet is in helping to identify specific foods or types of food which provoke a physical or behavioural reaction.

As standard allergy testing is best at identifying physical contact allergies, this can help to speed up an otherwise difficult process.

Conventional allergy testing typically uses a RAST test. This is a standard allergy test where varying dilutions of a substance – pokeweed, house mite dust, casein, cat hair, pollen or whatever else is thought to be the problem – are pricked onto the skin using a panel of small needles. It can identify contact allergic responses but is not good at picking up reactions to ingestion of the same things. This might tell you that you are likely to come out in a rash if you fall in a bath of milk but be unable to indicate how you would respond to drinking a glass of milk.

A further test that may be done is an ELISA (enzyme-linked immunosorbent assay).

A further potential benefit, where maintaining a diet with a limited range of foods, is trying to ensure variety rather than getting into a set pattern of using the same set of foods every day.

What is the evidence?

Food rotation is not a dietary approach separate from those so far discussed, but rather a way of ensuring that a restricted diet is easier to stick to. There have been no studies looking at whether this is in fact the case; however, being able to vary the diet intuitively seems a sensible thing to do, especially in individuals who have a habit of developing fixed routines.

Resources

A useful discussion of rotation diets as used in ASD can be found on the TACA (Talk About Curing Autism) website at: www.tacanow.com.

CHAPTER 14

Possible Problems which Can Present with Current Diets

As we have seen, there is a wide range of approaches that have been advocated and implemented by and with individuals who have autistic spectrum disorders, and self-restriction of diet is not uncommon. There are common features to a number of these and a range of possible difficulties that need to be addressed or monitored. Carbohydrate restriction is common to the various low-carbohydrate, high-protein diets, the simple carbohydrate diet and to casein-free, gluten-free diets. All of these diets significantly increase the excretion of calcium with a consequently increased risk of both osteoporosis and the formation of kidney stones. It is also likely that all of these diets will result in a significant drop in vitamin B1 intake unless this is supplemented, resulting in an increased risk of possible retinal problems.

Most low-carbohydrate approaches will result in transient tiredness as the body adapts to ketosis and production of energy from fats. In addition, without careful attention, calorie intake will also fall and persistent lethargy may result from this.

The increased use of nuts and nut butters specifically advocated in the simple carbohydrate diet can result in excessive copper intake. This is also possible on a number of the other diets discussed. Elevated copper levels can interfere with both liver and visual function.

An excessive excretion of oxalic acid will result from reliance on higher oxalate foods. There is an increased risk of kidney stone formation with higher oxalic acid levels, particularly if calcium excretion is

Table 14.1 Possible problems with current diets

DIET	Possible problems with this diet	Corrected by	Benefits
LC-HP	Osteoporosis Kidney stones Retinal degeneration Lethargy	Calcium supplement Magnesium supplement Thiamine (vitamin B1) Time – only a problem in the initial phase of the diet	Enhanced sugar balance Better cardiovascular function
Feingold	None known		Lowered inattention and fidgetiness
SCD	Osteoporosis Kidney stones Retinal degeneration Excess copper Lethargy	Calcium supplement Magnesium supplement Thiamine (vitamin B1) Limit nuts and nut butters Time – only a problem in the initial phase of the diet	Enhanced sugar balance Better cardiovascular function
CF-GF	Osteoporosis Kidney stones Retinal degeneration Lethargy	Calcium supplement Calcium supplement Thiamine (vitamin B1) Time – only a problem in the initial phase of the diet	Enhanced sugar balance Better cardiovascular function
Low oxalate	None		Reduces risk if kidney stones Reduces GI and GU problems
GARD	None known		Reduces seizure risk

Table 14.1 *cont.*

DIET	Possible problems with this diet	Corrected by	Benefits
Low phenylalanine	Diet is low in omega-3 Diet is low in omega-6 Diet is low in carnitine	Supplement omega-3 Supplement omega-6 Supplement carnitine	Only of benefit in PKU or hyperphenylalaninaemic cases
Low phenol	Increased serum cholesterol		Not known
Body Ecology	Not known		Not known
Rotation	None		Reduces 'boredom factor' of limited food range on many of the above.

LC-HP: Low-carbohydrate, high-protein

SCD: Simple Carbohydrate Diet

CF-GF: Casein-free, gluten-free

GARD: Glutamate-Aspartate Restricted Diet

GU: genito-urinary

PKU: Phenylketonurea.

increased in tandem. Hyperoxaluria also increases the likelihood of painful urination.

It has been found that intake of high levels of calcium can reverse hyperoxaluria where this results from high levels of dietary intake of oxalates (Hess *et al.* 1998); this may not prove to be the case where there are other reasons for elevated oxalic acid such as aspergillus infection or a genetic condition.

PART III

THE SIMPLE RESTRICTION DIET (SRD)

CHAPTER 15

About the Simple Restriction Diet and Getting Started

The science of life is a superb and dazzlingly lighted hall which may be reached only by passing through a long and ghastly kitchen.

Claude Bernard (1865)

Trying to come up with a catchy acronym for this approach, the best I could manage was LOPGGATCSCD (the low oxalate, phenol, glutamate, gluten, aspartate, tyramine, casein and Specific Carbohydrate Diet). I somehow think the term 'Simple Restriction Diet' is more digestible and easier to remember.

If you have read this far and not skipped directly to this chapter, I hope that you will have built up a picture of the rationales which underpin the various dietary approaches we have so far discussed, and an idea of the importance of many aspects of diet in ASD and how views on these have been changing. These various dietary approaches all have their adherents and they all appear to have helped some people at the level to which they have been researched. The specific rationales for the various components of the SRD have been covered in the various earlier parts and are not further repeated here; turn back to the relevant chapters if you need to refresh yourself on the basis for any specific components of the diet.

Sadly, unlike a new medication that is under patent, where huge sums are thrown at proving efficacy, there is no mechanism to provide adequate levels of funding for research into these approaches, however beneficial they might turn out to be. No-one will make a fortune out of the benefits of people not buying or taking things, so despite the relative ease and practicality of adopting such an approach, it is difficult to set up and resource the research to prove it.

Without an 'evidence base' of controlled trials which meet the standards of scientific research required by NICE (the National Institute for Health and Clinical Excellence: www.nice.org.uk), SIGN (the Scottish Intercollegiate Guidelines Network: www.sign.ac.uk) and their various equivalents in the USA, Canada and elsewhere, dietary interventions will not be advocated by national organizations such as the National Health Service in the UK or service provider systems in North America who work with ASD.

It is a sad reflection on our society that it is relatively easy to research whether a new medication or artificial additive may or may not have unacceptable risks but not whether an exclusion diet is likely to have any problematic effects. As we have discussed, the outcome is that there is a lack of research in this area rather than a body of research showing lack of effect. In contrast, there is a large amount of 'anecdotal' evidence from parent accounts, pre- to post-intervention videotapes, and accounts from individuals who have experienced such changes for themselves attesting to benefits. Such accounts do not pass muster as 'evidence-based medicine' but strongly suggest the need for such research.

So, let's assume at this point that you are thinking of looking at dietary intervention. What do you need to do first?

As a starting point, given various issues, which we have discussed, it would be sensible to check whether the person who will be using the diet has any problems likely to increase the risk of having a negative reaction. As we have discussed, there are various possible factors that may have an impact on the likely success of a dietary intervention and which should ideally be checked out before proceeding. The first stage is to check whether the person to undertake the diet:

1. has diabetes (type 1 or 2) – evidence of problems that affect their ability to control blood glucose and ketones. This would not preclude dietary intervention but would impose a further set of restrictions and require careful monitoring throughout. Various of the approaches here have been advocated as

adjunctive support in diabetes care (see Atkins, Vernon and Eberstein 2004; Bernstein 2007; Ratnesar 2002)

2. has antigliadin or antiendomesial antibodies – this would be evidence of celiac disease, and therefore requires strict adherence to a gluten-free diet

3. has abnormal phenylalanine metabolism – if they have hyperphenylalaninaemia this may be unknown; if they have been treated for PKU they will be aware of this

4. shows evidence of mineral or vitamin depletion – various tests are available to assess body levels of both toxic and essential minerals

5. shows evidence of gut dysbiosis/yeast overgrowth/parasites. This can be assessed both from stool samples and/or by looking for metabolites, usually in urine; it would be suspected on the basis of gastrointestinal symptoms – bloating, excess gas, intermittent diarrhoea and constipation, nausea or vomiting

6. shows evidence of obvious metabolic problems – normally through urinary organic, and amino acid profiling

7. shows evidence of SCFA abnormalities – this can be done using either blood testing or a standardized rating scale of SFA deficiency (see Schmidt 1997).

Where clinically significant abnormal results on tests of any or all of these factors are present, it is important that the relevant issues are addressed as part of an overall package of biomedical care. Assuming that a careful clinical assessment has already been carried out, many of these factors may already have been considered so it may not prove to be as onerous as it first looks.

Is there a common factor?

One factor which is common to three of the approaches we have discussed so far is carbohydrate restriction – the Mackarness/ Atkins/ketogenic approach, the casein-free gluten-free diet and the

Simple Carbohydrate Diet all claim significant success rates in improving various aspects of behaviour and development in ASD. All result in the person using the diet markedly reducing their carbohydrate intake.

The proponents of these various approaches propose differing models to account for why they may be of benefit. In practice, as they all limit carbohydrate consumption markedly, they can result in both ketosis (excretion of ketones in urine) and lipophilic toxin release (excretion of toxins bound in body fats).

Table 15.1 Common factors in current diets

	Reduced carbohydrate intake	Reduced toxin exposure	Reduced intake of not easily metabolized compounds (subgroups only)
Low-carb., high-protein diet	☒		
Specific Carbohydrate Diet	☒		
CF-GF diet	☒		
Feingold diet		☒	
Low oxalate diet	(☒		☒)
Low glutamate diet			☒
Low phenylalanine diet			☒
Low tyramine			☒
Low phenol diet	(☒		☒)

Lowered phenol intake can be beneficial for certain subgroups of those with ASD who, in addition, have a problem with phenol degradation.

Difficulties with the breakdown of phenolic compounds are also likely to result from going on a dairy-free diet as the diet will result in a galactose deficiency making phenol degradation more difficult. If there is clear evidence of a problem with casein breakdown, and a low dairy diet is therefore advisable, it would be sensible to provide a galactose supplement or to use slowly fermented yogurts as recommended by Gottschall for those on the Simple Carbohydrate Diet as those will provide a source of galactose from the lactose. Lactose (milk sugar) is broken down in the process of preparing the yogurt, to give glucose and galactose.

There appear to be two things that are helpful for most:

1. reduction of carbohydrate intake to a level where it stops being the primary source of immediate energy

2. reduction of exposure to pesticide and fertilizer residues, glycated and lipoxidated compounds, growth promoters, exogenous hormones, antibiotics and other toxic compounds such as artificial musks and alkylphenols (such exposures are the primary focus of the Feingold approach).

Many of the substances that appear under (2) above are lipophilic ('fat-loving') so tend to be bound and concentrated in liver and in body fat. If this were a major factor, then encouraging the release of glycogen and fats from body store by carbohydrate restriction would accelerate the rate at which these toxins would be removed from the body. This could result in a transient deterioration during the period when free circulating toxin levels increase. This would be similar to the transient deterioration seen when yeast overgrowth is treated, and toxins are released in the so-called 'Herxheimer' reaction.

If toxin levels prove to be the major factor, then periodic dietary induction of ketosis might be sufficient to maintain a lowered toxic burden, and this could maintain improvements. If, however, improvement results from some metabolic effect of ketosis itself, as has been argued for the use of ketogenic diets in epilepsy, then the dietary regime may need to be maintained with ongoing ketosis for continuing improvement to be maintained.

Low oxalate

Some high oxalate foods are also energy-dense sources of carbohydrates, though many are not. Higher levels of oxalates increase the likelihood of kidney stone formation. Reducing oxalate intake in tandem with decreasing carbohydrate intake is a sensible approach to minimizing possible risk.

As we have mentioned, a higher oxalate intake impairs the body's ability to derive energy from protein, so some limiting of oxalate intake is advisable when on a low carbohydrate diet in any event. As increased calcium intake increases oxalate excretion, calcium supplementation can be of benefit. Bacterial supplementation with *Oxalobacter formigenes* may also prove to be helpful once supplements such as Oxabact™ become commercially available.

Low glutamate and low phenylalanine

Low glutamate and/or low phenylalanine intake may also be beneficial for some. Detail on these additional factors can be found in the chapters dealing with the low phenylalanine and GARD diets. It seems likely, however, that although helpful to a small but significant proportion of people with an ASD, neither of these additional restrictions is likely to benefit the majority.

The role of CNS glutamate differences in some cases of ASD, particularly in Fragile-X syndrome cases, seems important, but the relationship between dietary intake and nervous system function is currently unclear.

The complexities of implementing a low-phenylalanine, low-carbohydrate diet in particular are such that this would be virtually impossible without dietetic support and should not be attempted in those where there are no metabolic indicators of likely difficulties with phenylalanine metabolism.

Low tyramine

Tyramine is a monoamine that has various effects but its effects are most obvious in increasing blood pressure and heart rate, causing physical agitation and anxiety if taken in high amounts. Tyramine is known to trigger migraine in susceptible individuals, often being brought on by foods such as broad beans, sauerkraut, unripe bananas, processed cheeses, and by alcohols such as beer and certain red wines (see Millichap and Yee 2003).

There is, in addition, an interaction between tyramine and the function of one class of antidepressants known as monoamine oxidase inhibitors (MAOIs), which can potentially provoke a hypertensive crisis. A considerable amount of research has been done on the beneficial effects of low tyramine diets, but this research has focused particularly on how they enable patients to be maintained on MAOI medication (Gardner *et al.* 1996; Shulman and Walker 1999; Walker *et al.* 1996). Research on such interactions between nutritional and medication therapies is an important and often neglected area (see Kaplan and Shannon 2007).

Low taurine

Taurine is a conditionally essential amino acid, exclusively of animal and bacterial origin. A conditionally essential amino acid is one that can be manufactured within the body but only at suboptimal levels. It cannot be made by infants, but can be made by adults from the amino acid cysteine provided there is sufficient vitamin B6, which is a rate-limiting compound in the conversion process. Ensuring adequate taurine intake, as it is predominantly an animal product, is a problem for breast-fed vegetarian and vegan infants and infants on vegetarian and vegan diets.

Taurine is added to many stimulant drinks to increase arousal and maintain an alert state, and can be reacted to badly by those with ASD when taken in excess. There are no concerns over overt taurine overdose or toxicity.

Taurine has not been shown to have any specific ASD effects; however, its general effect of increasing arousal and energy levels can exacerbate difficulties with attention, concentration and overactivity where these are present.

First steps

On the Simple Restriction Diet, we discuss taking a similar approach to assessment of possible dietary effects as was discussed in the Feingold diet chapter – beginning with a period of strict dietary restriction of likely reactive foods, followed by their systematic reintroduction. What is different is that this approach is initially more restrictive, and in addition to carbohydrate restriction, it attempts to test out the various possible problem factors individually.

An important factor is to try to ensure that there is no undue nutritional restriction resulting from the diet. Unless there is appropriate supplementation, and adequate nutritional intake is ensured on a low-carbohydrate diet, a variety of essential nutrients such as fibre, thiamin, folate, vitamins A, E and B6, calcium, magnesium, iron, and potassium are typically deficient (see Freedman, King and Kennedy

Table 15.2 Recommended supplementation

Supplement   Dosage (listed by age and sex where there are differences)

Age	1–3		4–8	9–18	19–50	
Calcium	500 mg		800 mg	1300 mg	1000 mg	

Age	1–3		4–8	9–13	14–70	
Selenium	20 mcg		30 mcg	40 mcg	55 mcg	

Age	1–3		4–6	7–10	11–70	
Vitamin A	400 mcg		500 mcg	700 mcg	1000 mcg	

Age	1–3		4–8	9–13	14+	
Vitamin B12	0.9 mcg		1.2 mcg	1.8 mcg	2.4 mcg	

Sex			Female		Male	
Age	1–10		11–51		11–51	
Zinc	10 mg		10 mg		15 mg	

Sex			Female		Male	
Age	1–10		11–51		11–18	19–51
Iron	10 mg		15 mg		12 mg	10 mg

Sex			Female		Male	
Age	1–3	4–8	9–13	14–18 19+	14+	
Vitamin B1	0.5 mg	0.6 mg	0.9 mg	1.0 mg 1.1 mg	1.2 mg	

Sex			Female		Male	
Age	1–3	4–8	9–13	14–18 19–50 51+	14–50 51+	
Vitamin B6	0.5 mg	0.6 mg	1.0 mg	1.2 mg 1.3 mg 1.5 mg	1.3 mg 1.7 mg	

Sex			Female		Male	
Age	1–3	4–8	9–13 14–18		9–13 14–18	
Magnesium	80 mg	130 mg	240 mg 360 mg		240 mg 410 mg	
Age			19–30 31–70		19–30 31–70	
Magnesium			310 mg 320 mg		400 mg 420 mg	

(Data adapted from Hendler and Rorvik 2001)

2001). This is very different from looking at the effects of randomized supplementation in the general population, who are not likely to be nutrient depleted and where the evidence to date suggests some positive and some negative effects from supplementation. For example, supplementation with antioxidants such as vitamin A and E appear to have a negative impact on long-term mortality while selenium appears to have a positive effect (Bjelakovic *et al.* 2007).

As well as ensuring an adequate level of energy intake, the person should maintain appropriate vitamin and mineral intake as outlined, particularly ensuring appropriate levels of the key minerals – calcium, zinc, iron, magnesium and selenium being of greatest importance – and of vitamins A, B1, B6 and B12.

Minimum appropriate levels of supplementation for these key factors would be as shown in Table 15.2.

It is probably most sensible, at the stage of thinking of using a diet, to give a high-dose daily multivitamin/multimineral supplement from a reputable supplement company (such as Solgar, Kirkman or Brainchild). To ensure adequate body levels of key vitamins and minerals, this should be maintained for at least a fortnight before starting on the diet.

Starting with the SRD

The only real voyage of discovery consists not in seeking new landscapes but in having new eyes.

Marcel Proust (1871–1922)

Before starting on the Simple Restriction Diet, you need to be prepared with plenty of the foods and drinks that can be taken, and a good working knowledge of what is stocked in local shops (can you get local grass-fed meat, wild-caught fish, fresh shellfish, pak choi?). It is surprising when you adopt this style of eating for a while and realize that there are no snacks that can be picked up from the shop at the petrol station and few in the corner shop. You need to be prepared and take foods with you that are acceptable to the person and allowed on the diet, and locate shops and markets that can supply your needs.

Try to anticipate the obvious difficulties – look at the eating pattern of the person who is going to be adopting the diet. Where do they have their meals and snacks, how easily will they be able to keep to this diet in those settings – if we are looking at someone who uses a school canteen, for example, how receptive is the school to adapting to the diet or is it already available? Could they take a packed lunch instead? How would this affect peer contact?

Are there situations where the person will be easily tempted – maybe they typically go to a fast-food restaurant on a Friday, have popcorn and soda when they go to the cinema, or have takeaway pizza. Can you think ahead and plan a way of avoiding problems or conflicts? It often helps to keep a diary of the situations where problems do arise – even with detailed planning no-one is perfect and there will be situations where problems crop up.

If there is a strategy in place before the problem arises it will be far easier to cope with than if you have to 'think on your feet'. Say, for example, the problem is with snacks on a three-hour rail journey. If there are no snacks available on the train that you are able to have, it is too late once the journey has started to do anything about it. If you had pre-planned and taken snacks with you that you could eat then the problem need not have arisen.

Ideally, before starting on the SRD, a proper baseline evaluation should be undertaken, covering the various medical factors highlighted at the beginning of this chapter, and collecting information on current diet, clinical history, current level of ASD symptomology and level of functioning in various areas of prosocial functioning. A basic history proforma and diet diary are provided in the Resources section. Details for constructing a behaviour diary are outlined in the next chapter. It often helps in identifying patterns to keep the diet and behaviour diaries separately and match them up after the recordings are completed as this can help to limit observer bias.

CHAPTER 16

Living on a Simple Restriction Diet

Luck favours the prepared mind.

Louis Pasteur (1822–1895)

Many of the ASD children I have seen clinically crave carbohydrates – frantically searching the kitchen cupboards for biscuits and crisps, relishing fast foods and takeaways. You would expect that shifting the diet to one that is high in protein and lower in carbohydrates would make this 'scavenging' behaviour escalate. Surprisingly, more typically the opposite happens. A higher-protein, lower-carbohydrate diet typically diminishes hunger, unlike a low-calorie intake diet on which most people feel perpetually hungry. This can bring its own problems as we have discussed – if the person is no longer hungry, it can be more difficult to maintain an appropriate level of nutritional intake, and there will be an initial period of increased tiredness as the body adapts to using glycerol from triglycerides to produce glucose for energy.

The frantic searching for food we so often see is partly due to carbohydrate craving (Heller and Heller 1997) and partly due to the addictive nature of glutamate – many of the craved foods are high in glutamate, often in its stable MSG form, which makes foods compulsive to snack on. Although not well researched in ASD, there is some evidence to suggest that in atypical depression, at least, chromium picolinate supplementation can markedly reduce carbohydrate craving in a double-blind placebo-controlled study (Docherty *et al.* 2005).

Your body expects to have to work hard to extract energy from food because it is expecting to have to break down high-protein and high-fibre foods. When these are presented in an energy-dense pre-processed low-fibre high-simple-carbohydrate form, typically people consume too much energy for their requirements. It is no wonder that there is an 'obesity epidemic' with such a change in the pattern of energy availability and nutritional intake. (This is an oversimplification, but adequate for our purpose here. See Taubes 2007 for a more detailed discussion than is warranted here.)

Embarking on a Simple Restriction Diet requires considerable forethought. If the critical aspect is inducing ketosis, it is important to reduce carbohydrate intake markedly. Being aware of sources of simple and complex carbohydrates is important. Most people are surprised when they look at the carbohydrate content of foods like muffins and bagels, the varying levels of carbohydrate in different carbonated drinks (these can vary by orders of magnitude), and the levels in milk (high) when compared to cheeses (mostly low) – a little homework goes a long way.

The Simple Restriction Diet, if used as suggested and with appropriate support to ensure that there are no hidden problems which need to be addressed, is safe and can be adopted for many months, assuming the various checks and supplement suggestions are adhered to, with no likelihood of risk. This initial program has stripped out the major likely dietary culprits and 'cleaned up the diet' in a general way prior to working out a least restrictive beneficial diet regime. As it significantly cuts levels of refined sugar and carbohydrate intake, there are often benefits which come from containing problems with candidiasis (yeasts such as candida thrive on simple sugars, so when the levels of sugar in the gut are reduced, levels of yeast growth are markedly reduced) and improvements in complexion are often seen due to improved skin tone.

MATERIAL FOR TESTING KETONES

Unless the person in question has diabetes (where the key ketone, b-hydroxybutyrate, cannot be tested using nitroprusside urine test strips), ketones can be assessed using test strips which react to urinary ketones. In diabetes, blood testing is required and medical advice should be sought for the most appropriate and practical method.

Urinary ketones are tested usually by using a urine test strip, which reacts to the acetoacetate in urine. Various proprietary urine test strips are available such as: Ketostix™ (Bayer) (www.bayerdiabetes.co.uk), Combur-test/Chemstrip (Roche) (www.roche.com/prod_diag_combur.htm)

and Ketostrips™ (pHion laboratories). In addition, Uriscan™ (YD Diagnostics) tests urinary ketones along with a variety of other parameters.

Putting it all together – assessing the effects of dietary restriction

Swallows certainly sleep all winter. A number of them conglobulate together by flying round and round, and then all in a heap throw themselves under water, and lye in the bed of a river.

Samuel Johnson (Boswell, 1799)

If I have ever made any valuable discoveries, it has been owing more to patient attention, than to any other talent.

Isaac Newton (1642–1727)

Look at what is actually there, not what you are hoping for – try to be as objective as you can.

A first rule is to look at what is there and not to make assumptions about what you think might be happening. It is important to keep accurate records of behaviour so that you are clear that effects are real rather than hoped for.

Johnson's conglobulating underwater swallows were his guess about what swallows might be doing when they disappear from British skies in winter, but he hadn't looked to see if he was right. In the past, people have been absolutely convinced of ideas which we now dismiss – that the solar system revolves around the earth, that the world is flat and you could fall off the edge if you go too far, that flight is impossible in heavier than air machines, metal ships couldn't float, and numerous other things which were not backed up by evidence.

Public libraries have huge numbers of books on losing weight, looking like a filmstar, getting rich, building muscles, stopping smoking, stopping drinking and 101 other things. These tomes fill the shelves, and are typically well thumbed and frequently borrowed, not for the most part because they work, but because there are lots of people who are desperate to believe that they might.

I have lost count of the number of families who, when they see me, have already tried all of the remedies they have come across and have seen no worthwhile effects, because they have been all too ready to move on to the next approach before properly testing each one out. Often approaches which might well have worked had they been done well enough and for long enough have been tried for a brief period, and then dropped in favour of the next 'designer diet' or supplement with good PR.

As important as organizing and getting a dietary regime running is to work out whether it is making a difference. It should be clear from reading about the various approaches we have covered that in their full form many of these are not easily compatible, as one person could respond, say, to a low oxalate diet but maybe show no effects on a Specific Carbohydrate Diet, or vice versa. Working out what is effective for an individual can take time and needs to be evaluated systematically.

Preparation is nine-tenths of the game. If you have not monitored something you can't go back and do it in retrospect. Obviously dietary intake and amount of fluid taken need to be monitored. Try to make sure that you record information which is going to be helpful. This will differ from person to person – in one person it might be weight, searching for food at night, period pains and tantrums; in someone else it might be headaches, dandruff, constipation, dry skin and difficulties getting to sleep.

A baseline period of recording should give an idea of possible problem foods or food groups, dietary deficiencies and key behaviours or lack of behaviours. Remember that, for many people, those around them may have changed their own behaviour to accommodate – 'I never ask Jim to clear the table after meals because he always flies off the handle' results in a situation where the problem does not arise because other people have changed their behaviour to decrease the risk of Jim reacting. As far as possible, these other factors should be kept the same while introducing a change in diet, to rule out the effects of changes in expectation. If we change how we behave around someone this in itself will have an effect, so we need to try to take account of this. If Jim is now easier and more biddable, and we now start asking him to clear the table, we may see flare-ups in his behaviour, which are because we have changed our demands on him.

It helps at the outset to have identified behavioural targets – try to identify the primary areas that you hope might show benefit, things like:

- ability to learn new material
- retention of information
- self-care (dressing, toileting, caring for hair, nails, skin, eating and drinking)
- sleep–wake cycle
- bowel and bladder function
- obsessional traits
- stereotypies
- 'clumsiness'
- social interest
- aggression
- self-injury
- distress to loud noises
- 'other' (the various things which are specific to this person and don't figure on pre-prepared lists).

Having drawn up a list of behaviours which you are going to record, try to make out recording sheets which let you note down two types of thing about them. First record *what the behaviour looks like*. Here, it helps to record things like:

- How often does it happen?
- How serious is it (if it is handbiting does it irritate the skin, leave a mark, draw blood, expose bone)?

- How often for each incident you are going to record does it happen (if it is headbanging do they bang their head once, twice, three times)?

- How long does each incident go on for (does a tantrum last five seconds, five minutes, five hours)?

The second thing to record is *the situation in which the behaviour occurs*. These are things that psychologists often refer to as the 'setting events'. Here you would note things like:

- Who is present when it happens?

- What is going on at the time?

- Where does it happen?

- When does it happen?

It can also help to record things which you think the person can or should do but which don't typically happen. Looking for positive improvements – how often they smile, respond, talk spontaneously – may be just as important as how often they get in a temper. It is good to focus on positive behaviours as well as negative ones, but often it is the negative things which seem more important initially.

If the diet helps, it might cause changes in a variety of ways – things might happen just as often but for less time, fewer screams or bites or kicks etc. may occur, or both or neither. They might stop happening in some situations but not in others. Keeping good records is the best way of being able to establish whether something is helping, and, if so, what that something is. Keeping this type of recording should also help any health professional to see whether there are patterns that may or may not be food related – just because you have a problem with diet doesn't mean that you aren't also being teased, bullied or stressed for other reasons.

It isn't uncommon to review records and identify behaviour patterns that are linked to other factors entirely – additive effects of maternal PMT (premenstrual tension) can quite often show through in cyclical patterns recorded over several months, but are often not obvious to anyone at the time the recordings are made.

What can someone eat and drink on the strict phase of the SCD?

Reminds me of my safari in Africa. Somebody forgot the corkscrew and for several days we had to live on nothing but food and water.

W.C. Fields as 'Cuthbert J. Twillie', in My Little Chicadee *(1940)*

Diet

The aim in this first phase is to try to encourage the body to switch from relying on carbohydrates and simple sugars for energy to using glucose derived from three alternative sources: 1) from glycerol released from stores in the liver, 2) from triglycerides absorbed directly from fats in the diet which are freely circulating in the bloodstream and 3) from triglycerides stored as adipose tissue around the body.

There is no magic answer to the question of what should be eaten by someone on the strict phase of the diet. It will partly depend on availability – it would be pointless recommending cooking with Tef or Shirataki noodles if these are not readily available. This depends to an extent on the diet that the person has started out with – it helps to identify the lower carbohydrate foods which are currently being eaten during the baseline period. There may be foods that the person enjoys and which can easily be used as part of the diet; these foods can be seen as rewards during this phase.

In behavioural psychology, people often refer to 'the Premack principle' – if it is difficult to identify something which can act as a reward, look for things which the person spontaneously does, limit access to these, and use them as rewards – the person obviously likes them. With foods, the same usually applies, at least where the person has an element of choice. Given a choice of foods, we will normally opt for the things we like. If there are a number of lower carbohydrate foods which are enjoyed – say strawberries or melon – then these can be used as positives to help with the process of adopting a higher intake of low-carbohydrate foods.

Ideally, the person should try to adopt a diet which is high in animal proteins preferably from wild-caught fish, venison, if available, and grass-fed, organically reared farmed animals (cattle, sheep, pigs), and from crustaceans (although calves' liver and lobster should be avoided as they have higher levels of carbohydrate), good-quality eggs (preferably omega-3 enhanced), most cheeses (but try to avoid Roquefort and Italian hard cheeses such as Parmesan which have higher casein and glutamate levels). It is also best to use 'nutrient-rich' but 'carbohydrate-poor' vegetables (such as spinach, cabbage, kale, bok choi, peppers, broccoli, tomatoes, onions and celery) and fruits (strawberries, raspberries and melon). Cooking should be with olive oil, which is a monounsaturated oil, or canola oil, which is a mixture of omega-3 and monounsaturated oils. Do not use sunflower, safflower, sesame or corn oils which are omega-6 oils and pro-inflammatory, or coconut and palm oils which are saturated fats. High sources of glutamate should also be avoided such as soy sauce and 'marmite'.

By and large, be guided by the food listings which have been recommended through the book, in particular *The Calorie, Carb and Fat Bible 2008* (Kellow *et al.* 2008) for carbohydrate levels. This is helpful in giving comparisons across major UK supermarket chains and food outlets. Many of the sites listed in the 'further information on specific diets' in the Resources section also provide information which can be helpful at this stage. Other sources need to be consulted to try to limit intake of phenols, oxalates and glutamate.

Fluids

Drinks which are both sugar and artificial sweetener free are the best to take during this period. Water should be from glass rather than plastic containers where possible, to minimize exposure to plasticizers. Herbal teas, black coffee and green or black tea are all acceptable. All milk is high in carbohydrate and should be avoided where possible provided there is adequate calcium supplementation. Most fruit juices are high in carbohydrate, but lemon and lime juice can be used for flavouring.

Ketogenesis

So, having established baseline behaviour and diet diaries, and a programme of dietary supplementation as advised in the previous section, the next stage is gradually to reduce carbohydrate intake based on the general principles outlined above to a level at which ketosis is induced. This may take several weeks to achieve as many people with ASD have exceedingly high levels of initial carbohydrate intake, fixed eating patterns, and a limited range of alternatives. This can often take time and may also require advice from a dietician or nutritionist. Ketosis is normally seen with a daily intake of around 30 g of carbohydrate. Several features indicate that the person has achieved a ketotic state – there is a smell of ketones on the person's breath resembling 'pear drops' (a type of hard sweet); the person's urine also becomes concentrated and strong smelling.

Success in achieving ketosis should ideally be checked using one of the available types of urine test kit. These are widely used in checking diabetic control and are available both over the internet and from most pharmacies.

CHAPTER 17

Reintroduction of Foods

To safeguard one's health at the cost of too strict a diet
is a tiresome illness indeed.

Francois de La Rochefoucauld (1613–1680)

How do I test out what, if anything, is causing a problem?

Having used the exclusion plan as outlined, with appropriate
supplementation, and established that there is clear evidence of
improvement, the next stage is to identify what changes, if any, appear
to have been most beneficial in order that a least restrictive regime can
be introduced with continuing benefit.

At present, there is no hard and fast rule for how to reintroduce
foods. Assuming that you have used a low-carbohydrate, low phenol,
low phenylalanine, low oxalate, low glutamate approach and seen
benefits, I would suggest the following as a possible strategy:

1. Gradually increase carbohydrate intake, keeping
   phenylalanine, phenol, glutamate and oxalate intake low, until
   ketone levels in urine start to fall, but are still elevated
   compared to normal. Stabilize on this level of carbohydrate
   intake and record behaviour for two weeks. Assuming
   behaviour is as improved as before increasing carbohydrate
   intake, keep to this higher level of carbohydrate.

2. Gradually increase phenylalanine intake, again recording
   behaviour over a two-week period. Assuming behaviour is as
   before the increase, keep to this higher level of phenylalanine
   intake.

3. Gradually increase phenol intake, again recording behaviour over a two-week period. Assuming behaviour is as before increase, keep to this higher level of phenol intake.

4. Gradually increase glutamate intake, again recording behaviour over a two-week period. Assuming behaviour is as before increase, keep to this higher level of glutamate intake.

5. Gradually increase oxalate intake, again recording behaviour over a two-week period. Assuming behaviour is as before increase, keep to this higher level of oxalate intake.

   Given the increased risk of kidney stone formation with normal levels of oxalates and increased calcium excretion, a lowered oxalate intake seems sensible, but needs to be balanced against the level of dietary restriction imposed by this restriction.

If at any step there is a marked deterioration or change in behaviour or mood, remove the most recently reintroduced foods and wait for behaviour to return to the level seen at the previous step. Once behaviour is again stable, go back to reintroducing food groups, missing out the step that had resulted in behavioural deterioration. Once step five is completed, try reintroduction of any food group/groups that seemed to result in the previous deterioration.

If, as is possible, one important aspect of what has been of benefit has been the release of toxins bound in body fats, the maintenance of a lowered level of intake may be one key aspect to maintained improvement. If this is the case, sourcing animal protein that is preservative, additive, antibiotic and growth promoter free, and grass rather than grain fed, and sourcing fruit and vegetables that are low in pesticide and organophosphate residues will be important. Lower levels of exposure to flame retardants and phthalates from clothing, toys, and plastics are also likely to be important.

We have to accept that there is now a background level of exposure to various toxicants such as DDT and lindane breakdown products from which none of us is now able to escape (WWF 2007).

It is hoped that through using a systematic approach you will be able to identify a subset of foodstuffs that are problematic. If, as is most likely, a lowered carbohydrate intake is part of the best dietary approach to adopt, maintaining regular supplement intake is an important component of ongoing management to ensure good physical health and to guard against marked weight loss. The ratio of body fat to lean mass will change on a low-carbohydrate diet, and it may be helpful to monitor this using scales that compute percentage body fat and BMI (body mass index), which are now cheap and readily available.

How do I ensure the diet does not get boring?

If there are clear benefits from dietary intervention, the next step is to try to ensure that the diet is as easy to keep to as possible. A highly restricted diet can quickly become uninteresting, so it is important to try to ensure that as far as possible boredom with the diet is avoided.

There are four main components to this phase, which will be the longer-term implementation of an approach which it is hoped will be of continuing benefit:

1. Ensure that the diet is as interesting as possible.

   ○ As it is impossible to gauge what the maintenance diet will entail without going through the various challenge stages of the initial phase, I can't be prescriptive here. There are a wide range of recipe books and websites referred to earlier in the book that provide ideas based on the various restriction approaches.

   ○ This is where the principles of the rotation diet become helpful in ensuring variety.

2. Ensure that keeping to the diet imposes as little social restriction as possible.

   ○ If the person has a social life which revolves around going to cafes or other settings where control over food and drink is impossible, keeping strictly to a diet which does not allow them to eat or drink anything when you are there will be difficult, if not impossible. Being clear headed, problem free but socially isolated is probably not a net gain for the person concerned.

- Again this is where homework and pre-planning can be the most helpful – knowing the carbohydrate level in a portion of cheese and oatcakes, olives or carrot sticks as opposed to a muffin, bagel or panini can help guide food choice. What can you have and stay within your limits? Assuming that dietary challenge (see below) does not result in an acute regression, regular 'diet holidays' may be possible, minimizing difficulties for situations like vacations, respite breaks, celebrations, etc.

- Many restaurants, cafes and food chains will now cater to the special dietary needs of people when they are aware of those needs. The important thing here is to ask/agitate. Many of the major fast-food chains have introduced 'healthy' food options in response to customer pressure. The strongest pressure is a perceived customer base that is not being catered for. The increased awareness of celiac disease, gluten sensitivity, diabetes, ASD and ADHD has made this an important market force for which the food manufacturers and distributors will be eager to cater. By doing so they develop a USP (unique selling point), which gives them a market advantage – use this to your advantage.

How can I be sure that the diet is still required?

1. Periodically review benefit.

- We are all guilty of doing things because when we do them we feel something else we want is more likely to happen – the lucky rabbit's foot phenomenon. Just because we do something *and* something else then happens does not mean that the something else happens *because* of what we did first. This is what has been called 'superstitious behaviour', confusing temporal priority and correlation with causation.

○ It is always possible, even if you have been very systematic, that improvements occurred due to other changes, which paralleled the food restrictions which were put in place (a move of house, someone leaving the school who had been bullying, a new teacher, job promotion etc.).

○ It is sensible to review periodically the benefits which were attributed to the diet and whether these have been maintained, have slipped back or have continued to improve. When doing this go back to the methods which were used during the baseline phase, always assuming that these are still developmentally appropriate – try to compare like with like.

2. Dietary challenge.

○ In some cases, removal of factors which have been causing problems may have allowed the body to repair itself – reduction in intake of pro-inflammatory compounds such as omega-6 oils, for example, may have reduced gastric inflammation and allowed GI function to improve. Another case would be where ketogenesis had allowed release of lipophilic toxins from adipose (fatty) tissue and was no longer required as the process had removed excess toxins. In these cases, the diet may have been necessary for the improvement to occur, but may not be required for maintenance of benefits. In either case, reverting to the baseline diet may not cause problems; however, there is the possibility of a gradual development of inflammatory GI responses and of the renewed build-up of toxins.

○ Dietary challenge may be beneficial in indicating whether there is an acute response to reintroduction of problematic foods, or whether the reaction is insidious. In the latter case, periodic 'diet holidays' may be introduced without negative effects, as periods 'on diet' would enable self-repair to correct any build-up of potentially damaging effects.

- There will obviously be certain situations where dietary challenge would impose significant risk to the individual (as in individuals when introduction of the diet had resolved problems with suicidal thoughts, severe self-injury or aggression). In such cases, maintenance of improvement would outweigh the benefit of establishing a link.

CHAPTER 18

How Long Is Long Enough to Give Benefits?

'How long does getting thin take?' Pooh asked anxiously.

A.A. Milne (1882–1956)

As has been stressed at several points in the book so far, there are a large number of possible reasons for ASD, some of which are largely environmental, some epigenetic, some an interplay of environmental and genetic factors, and some largely genetic in origin. The different causes will lead to differences in how rapidly any change is likely to be seen and in how amenable the condition will be to change.

The length of time required to see whether a dietary approach is likely to be beneficial is largely dependent on the nature of the problem and on what is being tried. It is also important to have baseline information on the areas where improvements may be seen, as outlined in the last chapter, in order to assess any benefits.

If you are going to adopt the strategy outlined in the 'chronology for dietary intervention' in the Resources section, it will take at least 16 weeks to run through the diet and the subsequent food reintroductions, testing out the effects of varying dietary intake of carbohydrate, phenylalanine, phenol, glutamate and oxalate levels.

It has to be remembered that all treatments have a 'placebo' component to them whether there is an active component to why they might work or not (Bausell 2007; Evans 2003), and there may be effects on behaviour and development which are real but unrelated to dietary change. Having to be stricter over foods may be part of a general change in limit setting, which may result in improvements in behaviour. If you are documenting behaviours, this may have an effect on how they are reacted to, and make them happen more or less often – if instead of trying to deal with a behaviour the reaction is to note it down, this can have an effect on behaviours which are 'attention-seeking'.

Putting these additional factors to one side, what sort of timeframe is realistic in looking for changes resulting from a change in diet?

Low-carbohydrate approaches

A Mackarness-type high-protein low-carbohydrate diet should show detectable evidence (ketones appearing in urine) within a week of starting the diet. This is a clear indication that the body has shifted from using carbohydrate to using fats as its primary source of energy. It does not show that the diet is likely to improve behaviour, but it does indicate, assuming the model is correct, that the metabolic process required for ketogenesis to work is coming into play as an active component of treatment. If, as we have discussed, improvements are a consequence of toxin release, which may parallel ketone production, then the effects may be fairly rapid but plateau.

Ketogenic diet

The only study to date that has looked at the effects of a modified ketogenic approach with ASD (Evangeliou *et al.* 2003) looked at outcome at the end of a six-month period. The children who completed the trial had had four-week periods on diet, alternating with two-week periods off-diet. The most successful outcomes were noted in the children who had milder ASD symptomology at the outset of therapy.

PUFA supplementation

A simple method for assessing the benefit of PUFA supplementation is to use a rating scale that quantifies physical features consistent with deficiency. As with much else, the person with a PUFA deficiency may not show a 'full house' of features – it makes sense to contruct a checklist based on the more obvious features which are typically present (wound healing and infection rate are unlikely to be helpful measures unless either is a frequent problem – wound healing could be helpful in someone with regular biting as a form of self-injury).

A range of features can be indications of PUFA deficiency, such as:

- dry skin
- dandruff
- frequent urination
- irritability
- attention deficit
- soft nails
- 'alligator skin'
- allergies
- lowered immunity
- weakness
- fatigue
- dry, unmanageable hair
- excessive thirst
- brittle, easily frayed nails
- hyperactivity
- 'chicken skin' on backs of arms
- dry eyes
- learning problems
- poor wound healing
- frequent infections
- patches of pale skin on cheeks
- cracked skin on heels or fingertips.

See Schmidt (1997).

Where benefit is seen from PUFA supplementation, this is normally within weeks of commencing supplementation. For further information on studies which have assessed supplementation, see www.equazen.com/default.aspx?pid=145.

Low oxalate diets

If a low oxalate component to the diet or probiotic supplementation is used to reduce oxalic acid production, a significant reduction should be seen in oxalic acid levels in urine. These should be detectable within a few weeks of beginning the diet/supplements.

CF-GF diets

It has been argued that the effects of casein and gluten exclusion on body opioid burden will be different. As casein derived opioids are largely hydrophilic (water soluble) they should be excreted rapidly from the body – effects of a casein exclusion diet would thus show up rapidly in someone who lacked only the enzymes to metabolize casein. As, in contrast, gluteomorphins are lipophilic (fat soluble), they are bound in body fat and would take appreciably longer to be removed. This view is supported by research from the University of Sunderland (Whiteley *et al.* 1999). In this longitudinal research caseomorphins rapidly disappeared from urine on removal of milk from the diet, while appreciable amounts of gluteomorphins were still being detected some six months after gluten removal.

As we have discussed, various groups have produced contrasting claims concerning the opioid model and currently the issue is open to debate (see Cass *et al.* 2008; Hunter *et al.* 2003; Wright *et al.* 2005).

The increasing body of evidence does not wholly support the 'opioid model', as currently defined. From the literature to date, and parental reports, there do appear to be definite benefits from CF-GF diets. Alternative mechanisms would now seem to be required to account for these reported improvements which may, as has been argued here, result from factors such as carbohydrate restriction, ketosis, and/or toxin release.

CHAPTER 19

Summing Up

Nature is nowhere accustomed more openly to display her secret mysteries than in cases where she shows traces of her workings apart from the beaten path.

Letter from Dr William Harvey to the Dutch physician Dr John Vlackveld of Haarlem, 24 April 1657

In general:

1. Approaches that induce ketosis have been reported as having beneficial effects in a significant proportion of those with ASD, in control of seizure activity in those with various types of epilepsy, in improving various aspects of cardiovascular function, and in stabilizing blood sugar level in both type 1 and type 2 diabetes.

2. Despite expectations, both high-fat low-carbohydrate and high-protein low-carbohydrate diets appear to have consistently beneficial effects on lipid profiles (Luscombe-Marsh *et al.* 2005).

3. Ketosis can be induced by restriction of energy intake from carbohydrates, while maintaining energy intake from proteins and fats.

4. A number of factors need to be carefully monitored and modified during such approaches; in particular, levels of minerals such as calcium, magnesium, iron and zinc need to be maintained, and levels of oxalate containing foodstuffs need to be limited.

5. It would be sensible to introduce a gradual, basic, exercise regime, tailored to the fitness level and capabilities of the individual in parallel with dietary intervention to encourage more rapid utilization of glycerol.

6. Nutritional intake needs to be maintained to prevent excessive weight loss.

I hope that by now it is clear that there are a number of dietary approaches to ASD where the evidence, although not cast iron, is strong enough to make their further investigation worthwhile, both at the level of proper research studies and for the individual. The key features of these approaches are incorporated into the SRD.

This is a powerful approach to changing body metabolism, which can have both positive and negative effects, each of which has been discussed in some detail. In essence, this 'diet' has been used worldwide through the course of evolution and is thought to have been the predominant dietary pattern for most hunter-gatherer civilizations across the world; it is the diet which as a species we evolved to digest in all ecological niches in which we have thrived from the equator to the poles.

There are sufficient similarities in the dietary changes which are required by the high-protein, low-carbohydrate, ketogenic, SCD and CF-GF approaches, and in the effects of both cholesterol and SCFA supplementation, that all could conceivably be producing improvements for the same basic metabolic reasons – a reduction in carbohydrate load on the body coupled with better cell membrane integrity from an improved dietary phospholipid profile, and shedding of lipophilic toxins. If this turns out to be the case, then a high proportion of people with ASD may benefit from the same general approach, due to correcting aspects of the same common underlying mechanism.

There are at least two possible primary reasons that such a dietary approach may produce benefit:

1. Ketosis in and of itself may have beneficial effects on brain and body function – mechanism currently unknown.

2. That through inducing ketosis improvements occur due to the release of fat-loving (lipophilic) toxins.

If the first of these mechanisms is the basis for improvement, this dietary approach, once stabilized, would need to be maintained to sustain improvement. If, however, the problem is one of build-up of toxins, then the periodic use of this approach should prevent build-up and, once clearance has been established, prevent reaccumulation.

This view of ASD also provides a common explanatory mechanism that goes some way to understanding the link between ASD and a number of common comorbidities such as gastrointestinal problems, diabetes, anxiety problems and epilepsy, the co-occurrence of which with ASD is currently unexplained.

The evidence, viewed from this perspective, adds weight to the urgency with which the research agenda, highlighted in the MRC research review published in 2001, needs to be pursued. I hope that the various studies which are currently underway in Scandinavia and the USA (such as the MoBA, CHARGE and MARBLES studies), and the CANDAA study in the UK, will help to address the issues. Although confining its coverage to discussion of the casein- and gluten-free diet, the MRC review concluded:

> Although it is possible to provide a plausible biological hypothesis to explain the possible beneficial effects of gluten and casein free diets in ASDs there are to date no properly controlled studies described in peer-reviewed journals. Given the publicity surrounding these reports and, if substantiated, the potential widespread benefits, it is important that properly controlled studies should be undertaken to clarify the situation. (MRC 2001, Paragraph 140)

If a significant proportion of those with ASD can be helped to achieve a better quality of life through the adoption of such simple, inexpensive dietary means, this will be of enormous benefit to the individuals, their families, clinical services, and will significantly reduce the drain on government coffers (Knapp, Romeo and Beecham 2007). As these approaches are largely safe and resource neutral, we should be acting now and working out why they work alongside this simple and potentially significant development in care. We should not be waiting for the research evidence on the minutiae of why they work to come in first. For many families, this is happening anyway but is largely being ignored by the clinical and research community (see 'Families use dietary interventions whatever the clinical recommendations or admonitions' in Chapter 1).

To paraphrase the introductory quote from Gabriela Mistral: 'The child cannot wait, we need to act now'.

Assessment, follow-up and support

As indicated at several points in the book so far, it is important that the person who is going to undertake the diet has been assessed properly:

- to ensure that there are no contraindications
- to correct factors such as undermineralization prior to commencing a diet
- to provide an adequate behavioural and dietary baseline.

It is also important that appropriate professional support is sought to ensure:

- that response to intervention is monitored
- that changes to the diet are appropriate
- that calorific intake, vitamin and mineral content is adequate
- that there is no condition that contraindicates adopting this type of approach such as a liver problem or abnormal lipid profile.

As a starting point, it is helpful to note down a basic background overview of the person for whom the intervention is going to be tried, and the history of approaches to date. The 'background history form' in the Resources section should help to provide a rough outline, and save time when a consultation is sought.

A basic diet diary is also useful, although some components may be required to be looked into in more detail. Again some information on current diet will give a partial baseline.

For current diet, ideally a four-week diet diary would provide a useful starting point, but a fortnight before a consultation would be a useful starting point. It would be helpful if the foods could be looked at examining levels of the various potential contributory factors such as phenols, glutamate, phenylalanine, oxalates, tyramine, casein, gluten and carbohydrate. A variety of tables that help with this process are referred to in the Resources section, most of which are available as websites or downloadable pdf files. A blank food diary sheet is also provided in the Resources.

RESOURCES

Food Table

1) Possible reactive foods – if you see a reasction, this chart may help you to find what might be part of the problem. This is a selective list and further information on specific factors (such as phenols) can be found in 'further information on specific diets' in the Resources.

	Possible problematic factor in food							
	Phenol	Glutamate	Phenylalanine	Oxalate	Tyramine	Casein	Gluten	Carb.
Foodstuff								
Almonds		★						★
Amaranth				★				
Anise (licorice)	★							
Apples								★
Apricots								★
Artichoke								★
Aspartame			★					
Avocado					★			★
Bagel			★				★	★
Baked beans				★				★
Bananas								★
Barley								★
Beef		★	★					
Beetroot				★				
Beets				★				
Black beans		★						★
Black pepper								
Black tea				★				
Blackberries				★				
Blueberries				★				
Bouillon		★			★			
Bread			★				★	★

	Possible problematic factor in food							
	Phenol	Glutamate	Phenylalanine	Oxalate	Tyramine	Casein	Gluten	Carb.
Foodstuff								
Broad beans		★			★			★
Broccoli								
Buckwheat				★				★
Cabbage								
Calf liver			★					★
Cappuccino								★
Carambola (Star fruit)				★				
Carrots				★				
Cashew nuts		★						★
Caviar		★			★			
Celery				★				
Cereal				★			★	★
Cheeses		★	★	★		(★)		
Cherries								★
Chestnuts								
Chicken		★	★					
Chickpeas								★
Chicory				★				
Chocolate milk				★		★		
Coca-Cola								★
Cocoa				★				
Coffee				★				
Corn		★					★	★
Cornflakes							★	★
Courgette (zucchini)				★				
Cranberry sauce								★
Cream		★	★					
Crispbread		★					★	
Currants				★				★
Dandelion greens				★				
Dates								★

	Possible problematic factor in food							
	Phenol	Glutamate	Phenylalanine	Oxalate	Tyramine	Casein	Gluten	Carb.
Foodstuff								
Dill	★							
Doughnuts			★				★	★
Dried beans								★
Duck		★						
Eggs			★					
Egg noodles							★	★
Eggplant				★	★			
Elderberries				★				
Endive (escarole)				★				
Figs				★	★			★
Fish			★					
Flaxseed				★				
Fruit cake				★			★	★
Fruit cocktail				★				
Gooseberry				★				
Grapefruit								
Grapes				★	★			
Green beans				★				★
Gruyere cheese		★	★			★		★
High oxalate fruit juice				★				
Hot chocolate				★				
Ice cream			★			★		★
Iceberg lettuce								
Irn Bru (carbonated UK drink)								★
Kale				★				
Kasha								★
Kidney beans				★				★
Kiwi fruit				★				
Lager				★				★
Leeks				★				

Foodstuff	Possible problematic factor in food							
	Phenol	Glutamate	Phenylalanine	Oxalate	Tyramine	Casein	Gluten	Carb.
Lemon peel				★				
Lentils		★						★
Lettuce (not iceberg)								
Lima beans		★						★
Lime peel				★				
Mangoes								
Maple syrup								★
Marmalade				★				
Marmite		★						
Milk		★	★			★		★
Millet								★
Mint	★							
Miso soup		★			★			
Most seeds		★		★				★
MSG		★						
Muffins							★	★
Navy beans		★						★
Nectarines								★
Nut butters		★		★				
Nuts		★		★				
Oats		★						★
Oils								
Okra				★				
Olives	★							
Onions								
Oranges	★			★	★			★
Ovaltine				★				★
Pak choi								
Parmesan		★				★		★
Parsley				★				
Pasta			★				★	★

Foodstuff	Possible problematic factor in food							
	Phenol	Glutamate	Phenylalanine	Oxalate	Tyramine	Casein	Gluten	Carb.
Peaches								
Peanuts		★						★
Pears								★
Peas			★					
Pepperoni		★	★		★			
Peppers	★			★				
Pepsi								★
Pineapples	★				★			★
Pinto beans		★						★
Pistachios		★						★
Plums					★			
Pork		★	★					
Potatoes			★	★				★
Pretzels				★				★
Prunes					★			★
Pumpkin seeds		★						★
Quinoa			★					★
Rabbit		★						
Raisin bran					★			★
Raisins					★			★
Raspberries				★				
Red berries	★							
Red grapes	★							
Rhubarb				★				
Rice Crispies		★	★				★	★
Rice		★	★				★	★
Roquefort		★	★			★		
Salami		★	★		★			
Sauerkraut		★			★			
Sesame seeds		★		★				
Shrimp paste		★			★			

	Possible problematic factor in food							
	Phenol	Glutamate	Phenylalanine	Oxalate	Tyramine	Casein	Gluten	Carb.
Foodstuff								
Soy cheese		★		★	★			
Soy drinks		★		★	★			
Soy milk		★		★				
Soy nuts		★		★	★			
Soy sauce		★		★	★			
Soy yogurt		★		★	★			
Spinach				★				
Sprite								★
Strawberries				★				
Sugars								★
Summer squash					★			
Sunflower seeds		★		★				
Swede (rutabaga)				★				
Sweet potato				★				★
Sweetcorn			★					★
Swiss chard				★				
Tahini				★				
Tamarillo				★				
Tangerines	★			★				
Taro				★				
Teriyaki	★		★		★			
Tofu					★			
Tomatoes	★	★						
Turkey	★				★			
Watermelon								
Wheat bran			★	★			★	★
Wheat germ			★	★			★	★
Wheat			★	★			★	★
Wholewheat bread			★	★			★	★
Wholewheat flour			★	★			★	★
Yogurt			★			★		★

A Chronology for Dietary Intervention

Background history

Is there any history that might be relevant? – dietary or contact allergies, migraine, autoimmune problems, Crohn's disease, ulcerative colitis, self-imposed dietary restrictions/cravings.

ASD diagnostic profile – ADI-R, ADOS-G, DISCO, other components of multidisciplinary assessment (speech and language, cognitive, occupational therapy)

If there is any indication of a specific relevant heritable condition (e.g. PKU, SLOS, Down syndrome), investigate testing.

'Psychometric' baseline

Baseline measures of current developmental level and severity of ASD as currently presenting – ideally getting assessments on standardized instruments such as the Vineland Adaptive Behaviour Scales (a scale which measures communication, daily living skills, socialization and motor development) and a measure of ASD symptomology such as the Gilliam Autism/Asperger's Rating Scale which gives a measure of current behaviour and should be sensitive to change.

BASELINE BEHAVIOUR AND
BIOLOGY IN PARALLEL

Behavioural and dietary baseline records

Is there anything which comes out of baseline food and behaviour diaries suggesting any sort of pattern/common factor (high level of refined carbohydrate intake, sugar, aspartame, red fruits)?

Introduce a graded exercise regime

Starting from the person's current fitness level, using a guide such as the US and Canadian Airforce aerobics system (Cooper 1977) to measure cardiovascular function and set exercise targets.

SUPPLEMENT FOR TWO
WEEKS BEFORE COMMENCING

Begin pre-diet supplementation

– calcium, magnesium, iron, B complex (as recommended for age, sex, size and weight: see supplement table 15.2, p.166)

BEGIN SIMPLE RESTRICTION
DIET (FOR THREE WEEKS)

Simple Restriction Diet

– Continue with supplementation as on the pre-diet phase (this will need to be maintained assuming a diet needs to be adhered to, at least through to the fifth challenge phase.

– Limit carbohydrate intake, initially to 30 g per day, avoid high glutamate foods, high phenol foods, refined sugar, milk (most other dairy products are acceptable, but care should be taken to limit saturated fats). Monitor physical effects with ketostrips.

FOOD CHALLENGES
(FOR UP TO TEN WEEKS
DEPENDING ON RESPONSE)

Food reintroduction challenge 1:
Carbohydrate (two weeks)

– Gradually increase carbohydrate intake, keeping phenol, phenylalanine, glutamate and oxalate intake low, until ketone levels in urine start to fall, but are still elevated compared to normal. Stabilize on this level of carbohydrate intake and record behaviour. Assuming no deterioration proceed to challenge 2.

(Only where hyperphenylalaninaemia has been identified and phenylalanine levels have been reduced)

Food reintroduction challenge 2:
Phenylalanine (two weeks)

– Gradually increase phenylalanine intake to initial baseline level, keeping phenol, glutamate and oxalate intake low. Stabilize on this level of intake and record behaviour. Assuming no deterioration proceed to challenge 3.

Food reintroduction challenge 3: Phenol (two weeks)

– Gradually increase phenol intake to initial baseline level, keeping glutamate and oxalate intake low. Stabilize on this level of intake and record behaviour. Assuming no deterioration proceed to challenge 4.

Food reintroduction challenge 4: Glutamate (two weeks)

– Gradually increase glutamate intake to initial baseline level, keeping oxalate intake low. Stabilize on this level of intake and record behaviour. Assuming no deterioration proceed to challenge 5.

Food reintroduction challenge 5: Oxalate (two weeks)

– Gradually increase oxalate intake to initial baseline level. Stabilize on this level of intake and record behaviour.

Maintenance diet

– Having established the level of benefit which can be achieved from the various dietary components which have been tested, a maintenance diet can be developed and used.

Depending on benefits found, consider further biomedical testing.

Background History Form

1. Information on the person who will be on the diet

   Name _____

   Date and place of birth _____

   Current address _____

   _____

   Phone _____

   Mobile _____

   Fax _____

   Email _____

   Names and details of involved professionals (this will vary markedly depending on age and extent of associated difficulties if any)

Planned pregnancy _____

Normal/assisted conception _____

Any infections/difficulties during pregnancy _____

Haemoglobin levels through pregnancy (if known) _____

Food cravings/aversions specific to pregnancy _____

Any birth difficulties

RhoGAM (currently RhoGAM Ultra-Filtered PLUS does not contain thimerosal, but in previous forms it did) – this is given in cases of rhesus incompatibility _____

Any perinatal history of note _____

Pre-, peri- or postnatal depression _____

Maternal age _____

Paternal age _____

Sex _____

Any history of

relevant dietary sensitivities _____

physical health problems _____

immune difficulties _____

gastrointestinal problems _____

celiac disease _____

diabetes _____

Diagnosis/diagnoses (if any) _____

Height _____

Weight _____

Known dietary reactions

Problems leading to trying the SRD

Diets tried to date	How long for?	What response?
Nothing	_____	_____
Casein exclusion	_____	_____
Gluten exclusion	_____	_____
CF-GF exclusion	_____	_____
SCD	_____	_____
Other	_____	_____

Supplements

What supplement?	What dosage?	How long for?	With what response?
Minerals	_____	_____	_____
Selenium	_____	_____	_____
Calcium	_____	_____	_____
Iron	_____	_____	_____
Zinc	_____	_____	_____
Magnesium	_____	_____	_____
Cobalt	_____	_____	_____

What supplement?	What dosage?	How long for?	With what response?
Multimineral	_____	_____	_____
Multivitamin	_____	_____	_____
Vitamin A	_____	_____	_____
Vitamin B1	_____	_____	_____
Vitamin B6	_____	_____	_____
Vitamin B12	_____	_____	_____

(oral/cream/spray/subcutaneous injection/intramuscular injection)

Vitamin C	_____	_____	_____

Enzyme supplements

Lactase _____

Caseoglutenase _____

V-Gest/No-Phenol/Phenol Assist _____

Other _____

Compounded amino acid supplementation _____

Galactose _____

Bacterial supplements _____

l-Carnitine _____

Yeast control agents _____

Antifungal agents _____

Other _____

2. Family history of

Relevant dietary sensitivities _____

Physical health problems _____

Immune difficulties (possibly migraine, systemic lupus (SLE), eczema, atopy, arthritis) _____

Gastrointestinal problems _____

Coeliac disease _____

Diabetes (type 1, type 2 or gestational) _____

Mental health diagnoses _____

Food Diary

Date

	Breakfast	Snack	Lunch	Snack	Dinner	Supper
Foods						
Drinks						

Date

	Breakfast	Snack	Lunch	Snack	Dinner	Supper
Foods						
Drinks						

Date

	Breakfast	Snack	Lunch	Snack	Dinner	Supper
Foods						
Drinks						

Date

	Breakfast	Snack	Lunch	Snack	Dinner	Supper
Foods						
Drinks						

Date

	Breakfast	Snack	Lunch	Snack	Dinner	Supper
Foods						
Drinks						

Date						
	Breakfast	Snack	Lunch	Snack	Dinner	Supper
Foods						
Drinks						

Date						
	Breakfast	Snack	Lunch	Snack	Dinner	Supper
Foods						
Drinks						

It may also be useful to monitor various physical parameters, such as the following:

Date _____

Body weight _____

Body mass index _____

% Body fat _____

Heart rate _____

Blood pressure _____

Urinary ketones _____

Further Information on Specific Diets

The Mackarness (low-carbohydrate, high-protein) diet

High-protein, medium-fat, low-carbohydrate diets

The Mackarness diet: a pdf file of the original *Eat Fat and Grow Slim* book can be downloaded from: www.cybernaut.com.au/optimal_nutrition/informa-tion/library/eat_fat.pdf.

A modified Mackarness diet can be found in: Hodson, A.H. (1992) 'Empirical use of exclusion diets in chronic disorders: discussion paper.' *Journal of the Royal Society of Medicine*, 85: 556–559.

A variety of internet sites that promote/discuss the various high-protein low-carbohydrate diet plans such as the Atkins diet are readily accessible.

www.atkins.com/ – this is the official site for the Atkins Nutritionals Inc.

www.carbwire.com/ – an online US magazine and discussion site on low-carbohydrate diets.

www.weightlossresources.co.uk/lostart.htm – a UK site with several more critical evaluations of high-protein, low-carbohydrate diet plans.

Information on carbohydrates in foods

A wide range of web-based resources are available, many through Atkins diet resources. One useful site is: http://lowcarb4life.sugarbane.com/lowcarbfoods.htm.

As it is often difficult to obtain specific information on branded foods and on the contents of foods obtained from franchised outlets, I would recommend again Kellow *et al.* (2008) as one of the most thorough UK guides on this topic, and Triumph Dining (2007, 2008) as an equivalent North American resource.

The Feingold diet

The best source of support on this as a specific dietary intervention is from the Feingold Association of the United States; their website is: www.feingold.org/index.html.

The Specific Carbohydrate Diet
Specific carbohydrate dietary advice

The Gottschall SCD as advocated for ASD is detailed in her various writings and the websites detailed under resources.

Her paper, Gottschall, E. (2004) 'Digestion-gut-autism connection: the Specific Carbohydrate Diet', is published in *Medical Veritas*, 1: 261–271. A pdf copy of the paper is downloadable from: www.breakingtheviciouscycle.info/news/Man261_271.pdf.

The CF-GF diet

A range of resources is helpful for those undertaking a casein-free gluten-free diet. A good starting point is the Autism Research Unit at the University of Sunderland, website: http://osiris.sunderland.ac.uk/autism.

The low oxalate diet
Low oxalate foods

The University of Pittsburgh Medical Center produces a useful handout detailing what are low, medium and high oxalate foods. This is downloadable from: http://patienteducation.upmc.com/Pdf/LowOxalateDiet.pdf.

The low glutamate diet / GARD (glutamate-aspartate restricted diet)
Low glutamate foods

Information on the GARD diet can be found at: http://dogtorj.tripod.com/id31.html.

The low phenylalanine diet

A number of hospital websites explain the PKU diet. The PKU Clinic site at the University of Washington in Seattle is fairly representative: http://depts.washington.edu/pku/diet.html.

The low phenol diet

Low phenol foods

There are a number of internet sites which give lists of high and low phenol foods such as www.zipworld.com.au/~ataraxy/Amines_list.html which provides a list of foods by amine level (a subgroup of phenols), and www.danasview.net/phenol.htm.

A number of phenol-absorbing supplements have also been developed; however, some reservations have been raised over possible problems with adopting this approach, and there has been considerable debate (see, for example, issues raised by Jon Pangborn at: www.autismtoday.com/articles/rebuttalrimland.html).

For a simple listing of phenol levels in different foodstuffs, see Seroussi (1999).

The Body Ecology Diet

Further information on the Body Ecology Diet and a brochure on the diet as applied to autism can be downloaded from Donna Gates' website: www.bodyecology.com.

The rotation diet

Various 'rotation diets' are in use. Information on one particular version which has been applied in ASD can be found at: www.specialfoods.com/rotationdietexample.html.

Glossary of Terms

β-hydroxybutyrate   A ketone body produced during ketogenesis.

3 beta-hydroxysteroid Delta7-reductase   The enzyme which is deficient in Smith-Lemli-Opitz syndrome and which is important in the production of cholesterol.

Acetoacetic acid   A ketone formed when the body uses fat rather than glucose to produce energy. This can be due to lack of insulin, which metabolizes glucose, lack of available glucose, or starvation.

Acetone   A ketone formed when the body uses fat rather than glucose to produce energy. This can be due to lack of insulin, which metabolizes glucose, lack of available glucose, or starvation.

ADI-R (Autism Diagnostic Interview – Revised)   A standardized scale which systematically enquires about areas relevant to the criteria used in the diagnosis of autism. Used by trained practitioners, it is recognized as the 'gold standard' for diagnosis.

ADOS (Autism Diagnostic Observation Schedule)   An observational assessment, developed to complement the ADI-R, which looks at current behaviour and rates current behaviour for consistency with an ASD diagnosis.

AGRE (Autism Genetic Resource Exchange)   A Los Angeles based international collaborative bank of tissue samples for genetic research, and matched behavioural and diagnostic data from large numbers of ASD families.

Alanine glyoxylate aminotransferase (AGT)   A peroxisomal liver enzyme. In some genetic forms of hyperoxaluria the enzyme is mislocalized to the mitochondria.

Alitame   An artificial sweetener, currently used in Mexico, Australia, New Zealand and China, but not in Europe or North America.

Alkylphenols   These are widely used chemicals – as plasticizers and ultraviolet stabilizers in plastics, as detergents (surfactants), emulsifiers, dispersants and wetting agents. Found as contaminants in both cord blood and breast milk.

Alpha-linolenic acid   A polyunsaturated omega-3 fatty acid. ALA is a constituent of vegetable oils, most notably rapeseed (canola), soyabean, walnut, flax/linseed and chia.

Alzheimer's disease   A degenerative condition which is the most common cause of dementia. Causation is complex but thought in many cases to relate to inheritance of the E4 allele of the alipoprotein E gene and in some an interaction between this susceptibility factor and herpes simplex virus infection.

Amaranth   The staple grain crop of the Aztecs, similar in carbohydrate value to rice and maize but gluten-free. Cultivated in Central America for at least 8000 years.

AMPA   Alpha-amino-3-hydroxy-5-methyl-4-isoxazolepropionic acid is a molecule similar in structure to glutamate but with selective action on ionotropic glutamate receptors, and no action on metabatropic glutamate receptors (such as mGluR5, the specific receptor implicated in FRAX).

ANDI (Autism Network for Dietary Intervention)   An organization set up by Lisa Lewis and Karyn Seroussi to provide information and support to families implementing or exploring dietary interventions for ASD.

Antiendomesial antibodies   These are specific antibodies produced by the immune system in response to gluten in individuals with celiac disease.

Antigliadin antibodies   These are specific antibodies produced by the immune system in response to gluten in individuals with celiac disease.

Aquaporin   A family of genetic factors important in water selective cell membrane channels. Different members operate in different somatic systems – aquaporin-1 appears to be erythrocyte (red blood cell) specific, while aquaporin-4 is CNS specific.

Arachidonic acid   A long-chain polyunsaturated fatty acid derived from omega-6 (linoleic acid), resulting in pro-inflammatory thromboxanes, leucotrienes and prostaglandins.

Arthritis   An inflammatory disorder of the joints, often thought to have an autoimmune basis. There are over 100 recognized types of arthritis.

Artificial musks   Artificial fragrances added to shower gels, soaps, hand lotions, perfumes, household cleaning products and certain foods. Many have effects on oestrogen receptors.

ARU (Autism Research Unit)   A research group, based at the University of Sunderland, which examines and researches biochemical aspects of ASD.

Aspartame   An artificial sweetener, some 150 times sweeter than sugar, with excitotoxic properties. It is 50 per cent phenylalanine by weight.

Aspergillus   A fungal infection, contracted by inhalation, which produces oxalates.

Aspirin   Acetylsalicylic acid. Originally from salicin, an extract of willow bark. It reduces headache and fever, probably by blocking production of pro-inflammatory prostaglandins.

Asthma   A chronic inflammatory disease of the lungs and upper airways.

Atkins diet   An American high-protein low-carbohydrate dietary plan for weight reduction and control.

Atopic dermatitis   Skin conditions, typically resulting in dry, thickened crusted skin. Thought to be triggered by immune factors and/or stress.

ATP (adenosine triphosphate)   A nucleotide which is used to create intracellular energy critical for the metabolism of all organisms.

Avenins   The gluten-like molecule found in oats.

Avian flu   Avian influenza/flu is a viral infection of birds which has, to date, shown very limited capability to be contracted by humans without close, normally blood-to-blood, contact.

Benzoic acid   A preservative added to many pickles, sauces and chutneys, found naturally in various fruits such as cranberries, prunes, greengages, and cloudberries, and also in the spice cinnamon.

Bisphenol A   A compound found in phenolic and epoxy resins.

Blood clotting disorders   A number of conditions which lead to abnormalities of blood clotting when the skin is cut.

Bovine spongiform encephalopathy (BSE) aka 'mad cow disease'   A central nervous system disease thought to be transmitted by a prion – a sub-viral pathogen. This can be contracted by humans through eating infected meat.

Brominated flame retardants   The most commonly used flame retardants used in furniture, clothing, material and electronic equipment since 1978. Some forms accumulate with exposure.

BSE   see Bovine spongiform encephalopathy.

Butylated hydroxyanisole (BHA)   A fat stabilizer and preservative used in fats and oils to prevent them becoming rancid. It is banned from use in Japan. Can provoke a range of physical symptoms including asthma, eczema, headaches and irritable bowel symptoms.

Butylated hydroxytoluene (BHT)   A fat stabilizer and preservative used in fats and oils to prevent them becoming rancid. It is banned from use in Japan. Can provoke a range of physical symptoms including asthma, eczema, headaches and irritable bowel symptoms.

Calcium   Symbol *Ca*, atomic number 20, a silvery white metallic element essential for the development of the skeleton and teeth.

Calprotectin   A calcium-binding protein found in the gut, which provides a biomarker for gut inflammation.

CANDAA (CAN Diet Affect Autism)   A proposed controlled study of casein-free gluten-free diet, based at the Nuffield Clinic at the University of Newcastle, currently trying to attract funding.

Candida   A group of yeast-like fungi which thrive in damp body areas and can cause systemic infections, abdominal discomfort and itching.

Carbohydrate   Sugars, starch and cellulose components of the animal diet. Not essential for nutrition, but a rapidly accessible energy source compared with proteins and fats.

Caribou   Arctic deer.

Carnitine   Derived from the amino acid lysine, carnitine is critical for the transport of fatty acids into mitochondria for oxidation.

CARS (Childhood Autism Rating Scale)   A standardized rating scale of ASD symptomatology developed as part of the TEACCH system used in North Carolina.

Casein   The primary protein found in cowsmilk.

Cassava   Also known as manioc, cassava is a tropical shrub. The root, once dried to remove cyanide, is a staple crop in many countries. Cassava is used to make tapioca.

Celiac   Celiac/coeliac disease is an immune disorder in which antibodies result in severe reaction to eating gluten-containing foods.

Ceruloplasmin   A copper-binding enzyme produced by the liver.

CF-GF diet   A diet which specifically excludes casein and gluten products.

Chamorro   A tribe found on the island of Guam.

Chemical individuality The notion, introduced by Archibald Garrod, that there were differences in sensitivities to environmental exposures, which would result in different biological outcomes for different individuals given the same events.

Cholesterol A cell membrane lipid found in all animals. Most is internally synthesized, and there is little correlation between dietary cholesterol intake and blood cholesterol levels.

Chromium picolinate Chromium is required in trace amounts by the body and is found in various foods such as carrots, potatoes, broccoli, wholegrain products, and in molasses. As chromium picolinate it is bound with tryptophan and has been shown to have appetite-suppressant effects.

Cirrhosis Progressive loss of liver function due to chronic disease.

Clostridium difficile Gram positive motile bacteria. More severe reactions are experienced by individuals who have poorer immune function.

Colorectal cancer Cancer of the large bowel.

Combur-test™/Chemstrip™ Several proprietary test kits for compounds including urinary ketones manufactured by Roche Diagnostics.

Cowsmilk proteins A number of proteins are found in cowsmilk (α, β and K-casein, α- and β-lactoglobulin, lactoferrin and transferrin).

Cyanide Derived from the Greek word for blue. Cyanide is a toxin found in cassava roots and cycad nuts, and in small amounts in apple and mango seeds and in almonds. There is cyanide in tobacco smoke and in the chemical form of vitamin B12 'cyanocobalamin', and in plastics derived from acrylonitrile. Cyanide toxicity: as a toxin, cyanide inhibits cytochrome C oxidase thus interfering with mitochondrial function.

Cyanocobalamin A chemically produced form of vitamin B12, which includes a cyanide molecule.

Cycad A cyanide-containing plant group, the nuts from which have been used to produce flour, particularly by the Chamorro in Guam, and which are found in the flesh of animals which consume them such as fruit bats. Ingestion can result in Lytigo-Bodig disease.

Cysteine A conditionally essential α-amino acid. It is required for the production of glutathione.

DDT DDT (dichloro-diphenyl-trichloroethane) was widely used as a pesticide from the 1940s until the early 1970s. Its toxic effects are still hotly debated but its breakdown compounds are known to have entered the food chain and be endemic.

Dehydration   Excessive water loss from the body. This can be due to a variety of factors including vomiting, diarrhoea, prolonged exercise, kidney damage and use of diuretic or purgative medications.

Diabetes   Conditions (type 1, type 2 and gestational diabetes) characterized by excessive urination where there is a problem with the ability of the body to control sugar levels due to a problem with pancreatic production of insulin or lack of a normal physiological response to insulin.

Diabetic ketoacidosis   A severe complication of type 1 diabetes due to severe insulin deficiency.

Diaita   The original Greek term for diet which had a broader definition, meaning 'way of life'.

Digestive enzymes   Enzymes in the digestive tract which function to digest macromolecules such as proteins, PUFAs and carbohydrates.

Disaccharide sugars   Sugars (such as sucrose and lactose) that are made up of two monosaccharide sugars (like glucose and fructose).

DISCO (Diagnostic Interview for Social and Communication disorders)   A standardized interview for diagnosis of mental health disorders, particularly focused on ASD, but giving a differential diagnosis.

Docosahexaenoic acid   An omega-3 oil thought to be important for the development of the eyes and brain.

Down syndrome   A developmental disorder caused by having an extra copy of chromosome 21, known as a 'trisomy'.

Eicosapentaenoic acid   A long-chain polyunsaturated fatty acid. This is an omega-3 fatty acid produced by the conversion of alpha-linolenic acid (from flaxseed, canola oil or walnuts) and/or docosahexaenoic acid (from oily fish).

Epilepsy   A pattern of repeated seizures, typically abnormal synchronous electrical discharges in part or all of the brain with behavioural sequelae.

Epsom salts   Hydrated magnesium sulphate, originally found at a mineral spring in Epsom, Surrey. Used as a purgative, but absorbed through the skin when mixed in bathwater as a means of improving the function of sulphation pathways.

Evidence-based medicine   Applying a standardized set of approaches to evaluating the literature in arriving at a 'conscientious, explicit, and judicious use of current best evidence' in everyday clinical practice.

Failsafe diet   A diet devised by Sue Dengate, an Australian psychologist, based on similar principles to the Feingold diet.

Fast food   Cheap convenience foods, which are cooked and served quickly.

Feingold diet   A dietary approach which concentrated on elimination of a range of toxins, additives and colourants.

Flame retardants   Chemicals used in the treatment of furniture, material, clothing and electrical products to reduce their likelihood of catching fire.

Flaxseed   A rich source of alpha-linolenic acid, a key omega-3 oil. Typically used as flaxseed/linseed oil.

Fluoride   Commonly added to drinking water to reduce dental decay. Fluoride is found in tea and in seaweed.

Folate   Vitamin B9, critical in the making of both DNA and RNA. Deficiencies in the first trimester (three months) of pregnancy can result in a range of birth defects including neural tube defects, cardiac malformations, genito-urinary abnormalities and cleft lip and palate.

Food refusal/avoidance   Where an individual deliberately refuses to eat/drink particular things. This can be an entirely behavioural phenomenon or can have a biological basis.

Fragile-X syndrome   A genetic condition caused by a triplet repeat expansion at the FMR1 gene locus on the X chromosome. It is associated with autism in a high percentage of cases.

Fugu   A type of 'pufferfish' favoured in Japanese sushi, which can harbour a lethal toxin, 'terodotoxin', thought to be produced by a bacterium, particularly at certain times of year.

GABA   Gamma-aminobutyric acid, the major inhibitory neurotransmitter in the central nervous system.

Galactose   A monosaccharide sugar derived from lactose in cowsmilk.

GARD (glutamate-aspartate restricted diet)   A diet which restricts intake of glutamate, and aspartate, which is biochemically similar in its structure and mode of action.

Gastroesophageal reflux   Chronic reflux of stomach acid into the throat.

Gastrointestinal difficulties   Involving the stomach, large and small intestine.

Glucagon   A pancreatic hormone, which increases free sugar levels in the bloodstream, and so has an opposite effect to insulin.

Glutamate   A non-essential excitotoxic amino acid, first isolated from gluten in wheat. It is found in many animal and plant proteins, and also functions as a neurotransmitter throughout the nervous system.

Glutathione peroxidise   An enzyme which scavenges free radicals and inhibits oxidation.

Gluten   The protein found primarily in wheat and corn, an immune reaction to which is seen in celiac (aka coeliac) disease.

Glycated compounds   Compounds produced by the non-enzymatic reaction of proteins with sugars.

Glycogen   The major storage polymer of glucose found primarily in the liver.

Glyoxylate reductase hydroxypyruvic reductase (GRHPR)   GRHPR is a liver enzyme which converts glyoxylate to glyoxylate reductase hydroxypyruvate.

Grand mal   A form of epilepsy in which the person experiences tonic-clonic seizures.

Hay diet   A diet developed by Dr William Howard Hay which emphasized a specific pattern of food combining thought to aid digestion and weight control.

Heart arrythmias   Variations in the rate, regularity or sequence of beating of the heart.

Heparin   A medication which reduces blood clotting.

Hordeins   A type of glycoprotein found primarily in barley and barley malt.

Hunter-gatherer   The term used for populations who subsist by hunting, fishing and gathering wild edible plants.

Hydroxybutyric acid   One of the ketones formed during ketogenesis.

Hyperacusis   Sound sensitivity.

Hyperdipsia   Excessive fluid intake.

Hyperoxaluria   When elevated levels of oxalic acid are found in urine.

Hyperphenylalaninaemia   High levels of phenylalanine in urine which can be due to a number of possible causes, specifically in the newborn: maternal phenylketonuria; in older individuals, it can be due to heterozygous phenylketonuria, transient deficiency of phenylalanine hydroxylase or of p-hydroxyphenylpyruvic acid oxidase.

IAG (aka trans-indolyl-3-acryloylglycine)   A breakdown compound from gluten, which is thought to be present in the urine of individuals who have problems with gluten digestion.

Inborn error of metabolism   A term introduced by Archibald Garrod, this now covers a wide range of genetic metabolic conditions resulting from an inherited defect in a single enzyme system interfering with the functioning of a specific metabolic pathway.

Insulin   A hormone produced by the pancreas which reduces free sugar levels in the bloodstream, and so has an opposite effect to glucagons.

Intestinal permeability   The extent to which the lining of the intestine allows material to be absorbed into the bloodstream.

Inuit   The preferred term used for the indigenous peoples of the Canadian Arctic and Greenland.

Iron   Symbol *Fe*, atomic number 26. Critical in the transport of oxygen (as a key element in haemoglobin) and in oxidation (as a key element in cytochrome).

John Radcliffe diet   A modified, less restrictive version of the ketogenic diet used for the management of epilepsy.

Kaschin-Beck disease   A degenerative disease of the joints and spine, found across wide areas of Northeastern China and Korea, believed to be caused by ingestion of cereal grains infected with the fungal infection *Fusarium sporotrichiella*.

Kefir   A drink made by fermentation of a starter liquid (historically this is thought to have originated in the Caucasus where various animal milks were used); kefir d'acqua uses a sugary water base such as coconut milk. The drink is produced by the introduction of a mixture of bacteria, yeasts, proteins, lipids and sugars to cause fermentation.

Keshan disease   A congestive heart condition caused by dietary deficiency of selenium.

Ketogenic diet   A diet which encourages the body to switch from using carbohydrate to fats as its primary energy source through carbohydrate restriction and increased fat intake.

Ketones   The three ketone bodies, acetoacetate, beta-hydroxybutyrate and acetone, are used by the heart and the brain as energy sources. They are produced primarily by mitochondria from liver fat cells when carbohydrate is restricted.

Ketosis   The metabolic state in which the liver converts fat to fatty acids, releasing ketones.

Ketostix™   A proprietary urinary ketone test manufactured by Bayer.

Ketostrips™   A proprietary urinary ketone test manufactured by pHion laboratories.

Kidney stones (nephrolithiasis)   Calcium deposits which form in the kidneys, often when the diet is depleted in calcium, thought to be related to the binding of oxalates by calcium in the GI tract.

Kwashiorkor   A form of protein deficiency malnutrition seen in children who are fed on a high-carbohydrate, low-protein diet. Described in central African populations.

L-2-Hydroxyglutaric aciduria   An inborn error of metabolism which results in subcortical damage and stems from a difficulty in metabolizing certain sugars including the monosaccharide sugar galactose derived from cowsmilk.

Lactase   The enzyme which hydrolyses the disaccharide sugar lactose in milk sugar to produce glucose and galactose.

Lactate dehydrogenase (LDH)   The class of enzymes involved in the conversion of glycerate to oxalate, and pyruvate to lactate, found predominantly in the liver, kidneys, striated muscle and heart.

Lactose   The disaccharide sugar lactose in milk sugar hydrolysed by lactase to produce glucose and galactose.

Lead   Symbol *Pb*, atomic number 82. A soft dense metal, which has various neurotoxic properties.

Leeches   Bloodsucking segmented worms with adapted mouthparts and secretory enzymes to prevent the blood clotting, and anaesthetic agents that minimize distress to the animal being bled.

Lesch-Nyhan syndrome   A genetic syndrome resulting in learning difficulties and an obligatory form of severe self-injurious behaviour. It results from a defect in the gene for hypoxanthine-guanine phosphoryl transferase (HGPRT).

Leucotrienes   Breakdown compounds from polyunsaturated fatty acids which are then joined to glutathione or cysteine.

Levodopa   A medication taken to address some of the neurochemical differences which develop in Parkinson's disease.

Limbic   To do with the phylogenetically older brain system structures that control emotions and behaviour found in all mammals.

Lindane   A pesticide which is used extensively around the world but is now banned in the UK, USA and Canada due to concerns over the effects of chronic exposure.

Linoleic acid   An essential omega-6 fatty acid found in most vegetable oils. The precursor to arachidonic acid.

Lipoxidated compounds   These are oxidated lipid compounds, found in many processed foods, that have significant pro-inflammatory effects.

Lytigo-Bodig disease   A rare disease of the Chamorro tribe of Guam, thought to be caused by consumption of cycad nut flour and fruit bats.

Magnesium   Symbol *Mg*, atomic number 12, found in most unprocessed foods. It is important in respiration and in binding excess fat in the gut, preventing absorption.

MAOI (monoamine oxidase inhibitor)   A medication which blocks the action of monoamine oxidase – an enzyme important in the metabolism of monoamines such as serotonin and epinephrine.

Marasmus   A form of severe malnutrition affecting all ages due to severely re-stricted energy intake.

Megacolon   An enlarged colon (large intestine), typically a result of prolonged constipation.

Melatonin   A hormone produced in the pineal gland from serotonin, which plays a critical role in controlling the sleep–wake cycle.

Mercury   Symbol *Hg*, atomic number 80. A silvery metal which remains liquid at room temperature. Used in a variety of industrial processes. Known to be neurotoxic and teratogenic due to a number of accidental exposures.

Metallothioneins   A number of proteins and polypeptides involved in binding and clearing heavy metals from the body.

Methylmalonic acidaemia   An inborn error of metabolism in which metabolic processes involving vitamin B12 and carninine have been affected.

mGluR5 receptor   A specific CNS glutamate receptor implicated in Fragile-X syndrome.

mGluR6 receptor   A specific CNS glutamate receptor implicated in Fragile-X syndrome.

Millet   The term is normally used for pearl or cat-tail millet (*Pennisetum typhoideum*), though several other millets are grown for human consumption. Millet does not contain gluten.

Mithridatium   A protective concoction against poisoning used from the time of King Mithridates until the 18th century.

Mitochondria   Subcellular energy-producing organelles found in all animal cells.

MMR vaccine   A vaccine to protect against measles, mumps and rubella. The MMR vaccines in current use are live, attenuated vaccines so do not contain thimerosal/thiomersal, a mercury-based preservative used in some killed vaccines to prevent contamination.

Myotonic dystrophy   A progressive genetic muscular condition in which the muscles relax slowly after contraction.

Myxedematous cretinism   A condition caused by decreased activity of the thyroid gland, resulting in dry skin and hair, and learning difficulties resulting from iodine deficiency.

Naltrexone   An opioid antagonist which blocks opiate receptor sites in the brain.

Neotame   An artificial sweetener some 10–13,000 times sweeter than sucrose.

Nephrolithiasis   Calcium deposits which form in the kidneys, often when the diet is depleted in calcium, thought to be related to the binding of oxalates by calcium in the GI tract.

NICE   The UK National Institute for Health and Clinical Excellence. A government-funded organization dedicated to the development of guidance on optimal healthcare.

Nitric oxide   One of the only known gaseous signalling molecules in the vertebrate body. It is produced by the inner lining of blood vessels and can be increased in inflamed tissue.

Omega-3   A group of PUFAs which produce anti-inflammatory thromboxanes, leucotrienes and prostaglandins.

Omega-6   A group of PUFAs which produce pro-inflammatory thromboxanes, leucotrienes and prostaglandins.

Opioid   A compound which selectively binds to cell surface opioid receptors.

Optic neuropathy   A condition affecting the function of the optic nerve or retina, this can be a consequence of factors affecting blood supply to the optic nerve itself or dietary deficiencies affecting retinal function, particularly vitamin B1 deficiency.

Organochlorine pesticides A number of organochlorine pesticides such as DDT and lindane, which contain chlorinated hydrocarbons, have been widely used. All people now contain some residues from such pesticides bound in body fat.

Organophosphate insecticides A range of insecticides such as chlorpyrifos which contain a phosphorus atom and which interfere with the functioning of the insect's nervous system.

Organotins Compounds also known as stannanes which combine tin and hydrocarbons.

Osteoporosis Reduced bone density resulting in an increased risk of fractures.

Oxalic acid A strong carboxylic acid derived in the diet largely from plants that binds with calcium in the gut to form calcium oxalate, which is excreted. Deficiencies in calcium increase the likelihood of kidney stone formation.

Oxalobacter formigenes A bacterium that is particularly adapted to sequestering and removing oxalates from the gut. It is particularly antibiotic sensitive.

Oxidative stress Any condition in which there is an excess of free radicals (oxidants), a lowered level of antioxidants or a combination of the two. Typically a process which increases with ageing and in a number of neurodevelopmental conditions.

Oxytocin A hormone produced by the pituitary gland which appears to be involved in breastfeeding, social behaviour and the formation of trust.

Paraoxonase 1 (PON1) A gene involved in the systems that enable the metabolism and excretion of organophosphates.

Parkinson's disease A late-onset neurodegenerative condition of uncertain aetiology. A number of genetic factors have been identified and a number of environmental precipitants.

Petit mal A brief type of epileptic seizure usually lasting between a few seconds and a few minutes, at most often described as an 'absence' or blanking episode. There is no loss of consciousness and the person does not appear confused or disoriented in the period around the seizure.

Phenol sulfotransferase (PST) The phenol sulfotransferases catalyse the sulfation of phenolic compounds.

Phenylalanine Phenylalanine is an essential amino acid that cannot be made by mammals. It is required for the production of tyrosine, dopamine, epinephrine and norepinephrine.

Phenylalanine ammonia-lyase   An enzyme that deaminates phenylalanine producing ammonia and trans-cinnamate.

Phenylketonurea   A genetic disorder in which the affected person lacks the metabolic processes to deal with normal levels of phenylalanine in the diet.

Phthalates   Chemical plasticizers used particularly to make polyvinylchloride flexible.

Phytonutrients   Antioxidant and immune enhancing compounds found in plants. These include compounds such as lycopene, terpenes, carotenoids, limonoids, and phytosterols.

Pica   The deliberate ingestion of non-edible substances.

Placebo effect   Therapeutic benefit with no apparent active constituent to the treatment being employed. Typically used with a control group as a measure against which to gauge the efficacy of an active treatment.

Pleistocene   The period from approximately two million to 11,000 years ago.

Pomo dei Moro   Early term used for the tomato.

Primary hyperoxaluria type 1   A primary genetic defect in oxalic acid metabolism.

Primary hyperoxaluria type 2   A primary genetic defect in oxalic acid metabolism.

Prostaglandins   Twenty atom hormone compounds derived from fatty acids with a range of pro- and anti-inflammatory effects.

Protein-energy malnutrition   Malnutrition conditions such as marasmus and kwashiorkor.

PUFA   Polyunsaturated fatty acids.

Purine   Purines are key aromatic bases that are essential in the formation of DNA and RNA.

Pycnogenol   An extract from Canadian pine bark.

Quinoa   A Central American grain crop.

Rabbit starvation   A degenerative condition noted in early Canadian trappers subsisting on poor quality protein.

Rett syndrome   A genetic condition caused by a defect in the MeCP2 gene resulting in a neurodegenerative condition with a clear pattern of progression.

Salicylates A group of proprietary analgesics such as aspirin based on salicylic acid. Salicylates are also found naturally in a variety of foodstuffs – in many citrus fruits, strawberries, almonds and tomatoes.

Salmonella *Salmonella enterica* is a species of bar-shaped gram negative bacterium that can cause a variety of illnesses, is typically contracted from food and can be spread from infected poultry and eggs.

Schizophrenia One of the most common diagnoses of serious mental health disorder which impairs thought, reasoning and perception of reality. Pathogenesis, genetics and prognosis are variable and uncertain.

Secalins The protein found primarily in rye, an immune reaction to which is seen in celiac (aka coeliac) disease.

Selenium Symbol *Se*, atomic number 34, a non-metallic element. Involved in preventing oxidative damage through selenoproteins.

Self-injurious behaviour Injury inflicted on the person's own body which can be deliberate and intended or obligatory but not willed as in neurodevelopmental disorders such as Lesch-Nyhan syndrome.

Self-restriction Deliberate restriction of diet to a small number of foodstuffs.

SIGN The Scottish Intercollegiate Guidelines Network. A Scottish organization devoted to the development of best practice clinical guidelines on medical topics.

Silicofluorides A salt of silicofluoric acid which is used in domestic water treatment.

Sleep disorders A range of conditions that affect the length, quality or timing of sleep, or the presence of nightmares or night terrors.

Smith-Lemli-Opitz syndrome (SLOS) A genetic disorder of cholesterol metabolism that is associated when untreated with learning disability and ASD.

Sodium benzoate This is a compound found naturally in a variety of fruits including apples, cranberries, greengages and prunes, and in spices such as cinnamon and cloves. It can react with vitamin C to form benzene and has been detected in unsafe levels in some fruit juices in both the USA and the Antipodes.

Sucrase The enzyme which metabolizes sucrose to produce fructose and glucose.

TACA Talk About Curing Autism is a US web-based parent-focused resource for information on alternative approaches to ASD.

Tartrazine   A bright orange-yellow food colouring dye which is used extensively in foods, pharmaceuticals and cosmetics.

Taurine   An amino acid derived from cysteine, it is involved in bile formation and is a transmitter involved in brain and eye function. Taurine is a stimulant and is added to many high-energy drinks.

TCA cycle (Tricarboxylic acid cycle)   Also known as the Krebs or citric acid cycle, this is where, in the presence of oxygen, a product of carbohydrate, fat, and protein metabolism known as acetyl coenzyme A is metabolized to release energy.

Tef   Tef is a grain that is carbohydrate-free and is now widely used by celiac patients with no apparent adverse reactions.

Terodotoxin   A fungal neurotoxin found in certain tissues of the pufferfish.

Tertiary butylhydroquinone (TBHQ)   A phenol antioxidant that is added to unsaturated vegetable oils as a preservative.

Thiamine   Also known as vitamin B1 and as aneurin. Severe thiamine deficiency is known as beriberi. Deficiency can cause liver and brain damage, retinal degeneration and damage to the motor nerves of the eye.

Thromboxanes   Compounds derived from prostaglandins, involved in platelet aggregation and in the constriction of blood vessels.

Trans-fats   Fats created by the artificial hydrogenation of oils, transforming them from liquids to solids at room temperature. These have been added to many processed foods, and partially hydrogenated fats were used as hardened vegetable oils and margarines. These are now little used in North America or Europe because of health concerns.

Transglutaminase   A family of enzymes involved in a range of bodily systems including the factor VIII component of blood clotting. Tissue transglutaminase production is the apparent basis to celiac reactions to gluten.

Triglyceride   The principal component of most fats and oils – an ester of three fatty acids coupled to glycerol.

Triplet repeat expansion   Triplet repeat or trinucleotide expansions are repeated segments of nucleotide basis (for example, CGG-CGG-CGG…is the base pair sequence on the X chromosome (cytosine-guanine-guanine) which copies up too many times – this can be anywhere from hundreds to thousands of times – in Fragile-X syndrome).

Tyramine   The amine produced from the amino acid tyrosine. Tyramine raises blood pressure and is found in a variety of foods.

Valproic acid   One of the most commonly used medications in the control of certain types of epilepsy.

Vanillin   A flavouring agent which can be artificially synthesized or extracted from vanilla beans, extensively used in foods, perfumes and pharmaceuticals.

Vegan   A person who has adopted a vegetarian diet excluding all meat, poultry, fish, shellfish, crustaceans, dairy products, eggs and honey.

Venice treacle   A 17th-century complex treacle/honey based on the mythrodatium, with a complex recipe of roots, leaves, flowers and seeds that was believed to protect against poisons and venoms.

Vineland Adaptive Behaviour Scales (VABS)   A widely used standardized scale for the assessment of language, daily living skills, socialization and motor skills.

Vitamin B1   see Thiamine

Vitamin B12   A complex cobalt-based vitamin which is found mainly in the liver. Deficient levels result in methylmalonic acidaemia. B12 is one of a number of critical factors in the methionine cycle.

Vitamin B6   Also known as pyridoxine, this is a water-soluble vitamin. Supplementation can increase brain serotonin levels. It is involved in limiting oxalate levels as a co-factor in the conversion of glyoxalate to glycine. Found largely in cereals, yeasts, liver and fish.

Vitamin C   Also called ascorbic acid, vitamin C came to notice in the early treatment of scurvy. It is a potent antioxidant.

Warfarin   A vitamin K antagonist and anticoagulant medication.

Williams syndrome   A genetic condition resulting from a defect in the elastin gene on chromosome 7.

Wilson's disease   A rare genetic disorder which results in accumulation of copper.

Zinc   Symbol Zn, atomic number 30, zinc is a metallic element. It is an essential element in bodily function, being involved in over 100 enzyme reactions. Found in a variety of dietary sources, particularly meat and shellfish, root vegetables and cereals.

Helpful Contacts and Websites

Every experience in life, everything with which we have come in contact in life, is a chisel which has been cutting away at our life statue, molding, modifying, shaping it. We are part of all we have met. Everything we have seen, heard, felt, or thought has had its hand in molding us, shaping us.

Orison Swett Marden (1850–1924)

APRIL
(Adverse Psychiatric Reactions Information Link)
Website: www.april.org.uk
Not ASD specific but a useful web-based resource which provides information on adverse reactions to psychiatric medications.

ASAT
(The Association for Science in Autism Treatment)
P.O. Box 188
Crosswicks
New Jersey, NJ 08515-0188
Website: www.asatonline.org
A US site that provides information and reviews of a range of research studies on autism assessment and intervention.

Autism Data Information Centre

The National Autistic Society
393 City Road
London EC1V 1NG
Tel: +44 (0)845 070 4004
Fax: +44 (0)20 7833 9666
Website: www.autism.org.uk/autismdata
A large searchable database of over 18,500 ASD articles with abstracts
which can be searched and results downloaded on a fee per use basis.

The Autism File

PO Box 144
Hampton TW12 2FF
Tel: +44 (0)20 8979 2525
Email: info@autismfile.com
Website: www.autismfile.com
A UK journal with articles about range of alternative and complementary
interventions for people with autism.

Autism Medical

Website: www.autismmedical.com/gateway_2
This is the website of the two merged UK charities 'Allergy Induced
Autism' and 'Visceral'. The site focuses on dietary, environmental,
gastrointestinal and immune system factors in ASD.

The Autism Research Institute

4182 Adams Avenue
San Diego, CA 92116
Fax: +1 619 563 6840
Email: media@autismresearchinstitute.com
Website: www.autism.com
A long-established organization and website, distributes a range of
materials on dietary, alternative and biomedical approaches to ASD.

Autism Research Unit (ARU)

School of Health, Natural & Social Sciences
City Campus
University of Sunderland
Sunderland SR1 3SD

Tel: +44 (0)191 510 8922
Fax: +44 (0)191 567 0420
Email: autism.unit@sunderland.ac.uk
Website: http://osiris.sunderland.ac.uk/autism
The ARU has carried out a range of studies on possible dietary factors in
ASD. The website provides a range of theoretical and clinical material and
links to other sites of interest.

Autism Speaks – UK
North Lea House
66 Northfield End
Henley-on-Thames
Oxfordshire RG9 2BE
Tel: +44 (0)1491 412311
Fax: +44 (0)1491 571921
Email: info@autismspeaks.org.uk
Website: www.autismspeaks.org.uk

Autism Speaks – USA
Autism Speaks
2 Park Avenue
11th Floor
New York, NY 10016
Tel: +1 212 252 8584
Fax: +1 212 252 8676
Website: www.autismspeaks.org
This is a US, Canadian and UK based charity which has funded significant
developments in ASD biomedical research.

British Dietetic Association
5th Floor, Charles House
148/9 Great Charles Street Queensway
Birmingham B3 3HT
Tel: +44 (0)121 200 8080
Fax: +44 (0)121 200 8081
Website: www.bda.uk.com
Useful site for locating dietetic resources in the UK, with a range of
downloadable pdf documents on foods.

British Nutrition Foundation
High Holborn House
52–54 High Holborn
London WC1V 6RQ
Tel: +44 (0)20 7404 6504
Fax: +44 (0)20 7404 6747
Website: www.nutrition.org.uk
Provide a range of useful material, many things available as PDF documents.

Consensus Action on Salt and Health (CASH)
Blood Pressure Unit
Department of Medicine
St George's University of London
Cranmer Terrace
London SW17 0RE
Tel: +44 (0)20 8725 2409
Email: cash@sgul.ac.uk
Website: www.actionsalt.org.uk
A useful website on effects of salt intake on blood pressure.

The Daisy Garland Charity
Email: www.thedaisygarland.org.uk
Website: www.thedaisygarland.org.uk/thedaisygarland.html
This is a British family-run website providing information and support to families wanting to implement a ketogenic diet with children who have learning disability and intractable epilepsy.

FRAXA Research Foundation, Inc.
45 Pleasant St.
Newburyport, MA 01950
Tel: +1 978 462 1866
Fax: +1 978 463 9985
Email: info@fraxa.org
Web: www.fraxa.org/

The National Fragile X Foundation
PO Box 190488
San Francisco, CA 94119

Tel: +1 925 938 9300
+1 800 688 8765 (toll-free)
Fax: +1 925 938 9315
Email: NATLFX@FragileX.org
Website: www.fragilex.org
These are two of the main Fragile-X organizations worldwide which
provide information and support.

www.familyvillage.wisc.edu/lib_frgx.htm
This is a US-based support site from the University of Wisconsin providing
links to a variety of national Fragile-X organizations and to family message
boards and chat rooms.

The GFCF Diet Support Group
PO Box 1692
Palm Harbor, FL 34683
Website: www.gfcfdiet.com
A US web-based family resource for people implementing a GF-CF diet.

GFlinks.com – the gluten-free page
Website: http://gflinks.com
A US link page to celiac and other gluten intolerance websites.

The Institute for Optimal Nutrition (ION)
Avalon House
72 Lower Mortlake Road
Richmond
Surrey TW9 2JY
Tel: +44 (0)20 8614 7800 (general enquiries)
Tel: +44 (0)20 8614 7822 (clinic enquiries)
Website: www.ion.ac.uk/index.htm
This is a large not-for-profit educational charity, which focuses on teaching
and dissemination of information on general aspects of diet and health.

National Society for Phenylketonurea (NSPKU)
PO Box 26642
London N14 4ZF
Tel: +44 (0)20 8364 3010
Recorded information line: +44 (0)20 7099 7431

Text: +44 (0)7983 688 664
Fax: +44 (0)845 004 8341
Email: info@nspku.org
Website: www.nspku.org
The UK PKU Society, providing detailed information and support for families who are coping with PKU.

Nutritionnutrition
Website: www.nutritionnutrition.com
A website run by a practising dietician, Zoe Connor; it has useful ASD links and downloads.

Physicians Committee for Responsible Medicine (PCRM)
5100 Wisconsin Ave., N.W., Ste. 400
Washington, DC 20016-4131
Tel: +1 202 686 2210
Email: pcrm@pcrm.org
Website: www.pcrm.org
A US organization with a good website which provides information on a range of food-related issues concerning health, vegetarian and vegan diets.

Research Autism
Church House
Church Road
Filton
Bristol BS34 7BD
Tel: +44 (0)20 8292 8900
Email: info@researchautism.net
Website: www.researchautism.net/pages/welcome/home.ikml
Autism Research (formerly the Autism Intervention Research Trust) is a UK charity set up in 2003 to carry out and evaluate autism treatments. The website holds a database of over 60 intervention approaches with three levels of information on each. The diet and supplement section currently reports that the range of treatments used is too broad to draw any conclusions concerning efficacy.

SCD web library
Website: www.scdiet.org
A useful web-based resource on the Simple Carbohydrate Diet.

TACA (Talk About Curing Autism)
PO Box 12409
Newport Beach, CA 92658-2409
Tel: +1 949 640 4401
Fax: +1 949 640 4424
Website: www.tacanow.com
A California-based charity that provides information and support to
families with ASD members.

The United Mitochondrial Disease Foundation
8085 Saltsburg Road, Suite 201
Pittsburgh, PA 15239
Tel: +1 412 793 8077
US toll free: +1 1 888 317 UMDF (8633)
Fax: +1 412 793 6477
Email: info@umdf.org
Website: www.umdf.org/site/c.dnJEKLNqFoG/b.3041929
A US-based charity which supports and promotes the needs of those with
conditions which affect mitochondria. Mitochondrial conditions are
significantly more common in ASD than in the rest of the population.

A Bibliography of Some of the Best-Known Books on Low-Carbohydrate Diets

(Listed in Chronological Order of First Publication)

Brillat-Savarin, J.A. (1825) *'Physiologie du gout, ou Méditations de Gastronomie Transcendante; ouvrage théorique, historique et à l'ordre du jour, dédié aux Gastronomes parisiens, par un Professeur, membre de plusieurs sociétés littéraires et savantes' (The Physiology of Taste).* A. Sautelet et Cie: Paris.

Banting, W. (1864) *Letter on Corpulence Addressed to the Public.* Harrison: London. First three editions sold 63,000 copies in the UK alone – also translated and sold heavily in France, Germany and USA. Fourth edition (1869) included letters of testimony from a selection of at least 1800 readers who wrote to Banting supporting his assertions and praising his diet.

Mackarness, R. (1958) *Eat Fat and Grow Slim.* Harvill Press: London. Issued as a Fontana Paperbacks 1961. Revised and extended 1975.

Donaldson, B.F. (1960) *Strong Medicine.* Doubleday: New York. Subsequent publication: 1962 Cassell: London.

Atkins, R.C. (1972) *Dr Atkins' Diet Revolution; Dr. Atkins' New Diet Revolution* (3rd edn). New York: Evans, 2002. Atkins, R.C., Vernon, M.C. and Eberstein J. (2004) *Atkins Diabetes Revolution: The Groundbreaking Approach to Preventing and Controlling Type 2 Diabetes.* Harper: New York.

Cleave, T.L. (1975) *The Saccharine Disease: The Master Disease of Our Time.* Keats: New Canaan, CT.

Gittelman, A.L. (1988) *Beyond Pritikin: A Total Nutrition Program For Rapid Weight Loss, Longevity, and Good Health.* Bantam: New York; (2002) *The Fat Flush Plan.* McGraw-Hill: New York.

Heller, R.F. and Heller, R.F. (1991) *The Carbohydrate Addict's Diet.* Signet: New York; (1997) *The Carbohydrates Addict's LifeSpan Program 'A Personalized Plan For Becoming Slim, Fit, and Healthy In Your 40s, 50s, 60s, and Beyond'.* Dutton Adult: New York.

Gottschall, E. (1994) *Food and the Gut Reaction;* (1997) *Breaking the Vicious Cycle – Intestinal Health Through Diet.* Kirkton Press: Canada.

Tarnower, H. and Baker, S. (1995) *The Complete Scarsdale Medical Diet.* Bantam Books: New York.

Eades, M.R. and Eades, M.D. (1995) *The Protein Power Lifeplan.* Paperback edition published 2000. Warner Books: New York.

Andrews, S.S., Balart, L.A., Bethea, M.C. and Steward, H.L. (1995) *Sugar Busters: Cut Sugar to Trim Fat.* First written in 1995, and updated and revised several times, most recently as *The New Sugar Busters!* (2003) Steward, H.L., Bethea, M.C., Andrews, S.S. and Balart, L.A., Ballantine Books: New York.

Sears, B. and Lawren, B. (1995) *Enter the Zone.* Regan/HarperCollins: New York. A number of subsequent volumes have appeared including: *Master the Zone* (2006); *The Soy Zone* (2001); *A Week in the Zone; Zone Food Blocks* (1998); *The Age-Free Zone* (2000); *Top 100 Zone Foods* (2004); *Omega Rx Zone: The Miracle of the New High-Dose Fish Oil* (2003); *The Anti-Inflammation Zone: Reversing the Silent Epidemic That's Destroying Our Health* (2004).

Ezrin, C. (1997) *Your Fat Can Make You Thin* (2nd edn). McGraw-Hill/Contemporary Books: New York.

Schwarzbein, D. and Deville, N. (1999) *The Schwarzbein Principle: The Truth About Losing Weight, Being Healthy, and Feeling Younger.* HCI: Deerfield Beach, Florida. Followed by: Schwarzbein, D. Deville, N. and Jaffe, E.J. (1999) *The Schwarzbein Principle Cookbook;* Schwarzbein, D. (2005) *The Schwarzbein Principle, The Program: Losing Weight the Healthy Way.*

Groves, B. (1999) *Eat Fat, Get Thin!* Vermilion: London.

Ross, J. (1999) *The Diet Cure: The 8-Step Program to Rebalance Your Body Chemistry and End Food Cravings, Weight Problems, and Mood-Swings – Now.* Viking Adult: New York.

Goldberg, J. and O'Mara, K. (1999) *Go-Diet: The Goldberg-O'Mara Diet Plan, the Key to Weight Loss and Healthy Eating.* Chicago: Go Corporation. Most recently, Goldberg, J., O'Mara, K. and Becker, G. (1999) *The Four Corners Diet: The Healthy Low-Carb Way of Eating for a Lifetime.* Marlowe & Company: New York.

Audette, R. and Gilchrist, T. (1999) *Neanderthin: Eat Like a Caveman to Achieve a Lean, Strong, Healthy Body.* New York: St. Martin's Press: New York, paperback edition 2000.

Gittleman, A.L. (1999) *Eat Fat, Lose Weight.* McGraw-Hill: Los Angeles.

Ezrin, C. and Kowalski, R.E. (1999) *The Type 2 Diabetes Diet Book: The Insulin Control Diet.* McGraw-Hill: New York.

Allan, C.B. and Lutz, W, (2000) *Life Without Bread: How a Low-Carbohydrate Diet Can Save Your Life.* McGraw Hill: Los Angeles.

Kwasniewski, J. and Chylinski, M. (2000) (English translation by Sikorski, B.) *Homo Optimus.* Wydawnictwo WGP: Warszawa, Poland (paperback). ISBN 83-87534-16-1. Available from: www.wgp.com.pl/index.php?id_s=149&id_j=en

McCully, K.S. and McCully, M. (2000) *The Heart Revolution: The Extraordinary Discovery that Finally Laid the Cholesterol Myth to Rest.* Perennial/HarperCollins: New York.

Cordain, L. (2001) *The Paleo Diet: Lose Weight and Get Healthy by Eating the Food You Were Designed to Eat.* John Wiley & Sons: New York.

Ezran, C. and Caron, K.L. (2001) *Your Fat Can Make You Thin.* McGraw-Hill: New York.

Hart, C.R. and Grossman, M.K. (2001) *The Insulin-Resistance Diet: How to Turn Off Your Body's Fat-Making Machine.* McGraw-Hill: New York.

Hart, C.R. and Grossman, M.K. (2001) *The Insulin-Resistance Diet. McGraw-Hill: New York. Revised and Updated (Paperback), 2007.*

Braly, J. and Hoggan, R. (2002) *Dangerous Grains: Why Gluten Cereal Grains May Be Hazardous to Your Health.* Avery/Penguin Putnam: New York.

Ottoboni, A. and Ottoboni, F. (2002) *The Modern Nutritional Diseases: Heart Disease, Stroke, Type 2 Diabetes, Obesity, Cancer, and How to Prevent Them.* Vincente Books: Sparks, NV, 2nd printing, revised 2003.

Smith, M.D. (2002) *Going Against the Grain: How Reducing and Avoiding Grains Can Revitalize Your Health.* Contemporary Books: Chicago.

Kenton, L. (2002) *The X Factor Diet: For Lasting Weight Loss and Vital Health.* Vermillion: London.

Mercola, J. and Levy, A.R. (2003) *The No-Grain Diet: Conquer Carbohydrate Addiction and Stay Slim for Life.* Dutton: New York.

Agatston, A. (2003) *The South Beach Diet: The Delicious, Doctor-Designed, Foolproof Plan for Fast and Healthy Weight Loss.* Rodale Inc.: Emmaus, PA

Bernstein, R.K. (2007a) *Dr Bernstein's Diabetes Solution: The Complete Guide to Achieving Normal Blood Sugars.* (revised edn). Little Brown: Boston. Bernstein, R.K. (2007b) *The Diabetes Diet: Dr Bernstein's Low-Carbohydrate Solution.* Little Brown: Boston.

Morse, J.S.B. (2006) *The Evolution Diet: What and How We Were Designed to Eat.* Code Publishing: Seattle. *A recent book by Gary Taubes, a science writer and correspondent for Science, provides a wealth of background and historical information on low-carbohydrate diets. It does not mention ASD or celiac disease but provides useful information on several biomedical aspects such as diabetes and cardiovascular function.*

Taubes, G. (2007) *Good Calories, Bad Calories.* Knopff: New York. (Published in the UK as *The Diet Delusion.* Vermillion: London.) *An invited lecture by Taubes, entitled 'The Quality of Calories: What Makes Us Fat and Why Nobody Seems to Care', which was given on 27 November 2007 at the University of California, Berkeley, can be accessed through the following link: http://webcast.berkeley.edu/.*

References

Abrahams, B.S. and Geschwind, D.H. (2008) 'Advances in autism genetics: on the threshold of a new neurobiology.' *Nature Reviews Genetics.* Published online 15 April 2008, doi:10.1038/nrg2346.

Accardo, P., Whitman, B., Caul, J. and Rolfe, U. (1988) 'Autism and plumbism. A possible association.' *Clinical Pediatrics*, 27(1): 41–44.

Accurso, A., Bernstein, R.K., Dahlqvist, A., Draznin, B. *et al.* (2008) 'Dietary carbohydrate restriction in type 2 diabetes mellitus and metabolic syndrome: time for a critical appraisal.' *Nutrition & Metabolism*, 5: 9. doi:10.1186/1743-7075-5-9.

Adas, M. (2001) *Agricultural and Pastoral Societies in Ancient and Classical History.* Temple University Press: Philadelphia, Pennsylvania.

Ad-Brands (2003) www.mind-advertising.com/us/index.html

Afzal, N., Murch, S., Thirrupathy, K., Berger, L., Fagbemi, A. and Heuschkel, R. (2003) 'Constipation with acquired megarectum in children with autism.' *Pediatrics*, 112: 939–942.

Agency for Healthcare Research and Quality (2004) *Effects of Omega-3 Fatty Acids on Lipids and Glycemic Control in Type II Diabetes and the Metabolic Syndrome and on Inflammatory Bowel Disease, Rheumatoid Arthritis, Renal Disease, Systemic Lupus Erythematosus, and Osteoporosis.* AHRQ Publication No. 04-E012-2, *Evidence Report/Technology Assessment* No. 89. Available from: www.ahrq.gov/clinic/epcsums/o3lipidsum.htm.

Agostoni, C., Massetto, N., Biasucci, G., Rottoli, A. *et al.* (2000) 'Effects of long-chain polyunsaturated fatty acid supplementation on fatty acid status and visual function in treated children with hyperphenylalaninemia.' *Journal of Pediatrics*, 137: 504–509.

Agostoni, C., Verduci, E., Massetto, N., Fiori, I. *et al.* (2003) 'Long term effects of long chain polyunsaturated fats in hyperphenylalaninemic children.' *Archives of Disease in Childhood*, 88: 582–583.

Agre, P. (2006) 'Aquaporin water channels: from atomic structure to clinical medicine.' *Nanomedicine: Nanotechnology, Biology, and Medicine*, 2: 266–267.

Aitken, K.J. (2008) 'Intersubjectivity, affective neuroscience, and the neurobiology of autistic spectrum disorders: a systematic review.' *The Keio Medical Journal*, 57(1): 15–36.

Akhondzadeh, S., Mohammadi, R. and Khademi, M. (2004) 'Zinc sulfate as an adjunct to methylphenidate for the treatment of attention deficit hyperactivity disorder in children: a double blind and randomized trial [ISRCTN64132371].' *BMC Psychiatry*, 4: 9. This article is available from: www.biomedcentral.com/1471-244X/4/9.

Alberti, A., Pirrone, P., Elia, M., Waring, R.H. and Romano, C. (1999) 'Sulphation deficit in "low functioning" autistic children: a pilot study.' *Biological Psychiatry*, 46: 420–424.

Aldred, S., Moore, K.M., Fitzgerald, M. and Waring, R.H. (2003) 'Plasma amino acid levels in children with autism and their families.' *Journal of Autism and Developmental Disorders*, 33(1): 93–97.

Allport, S. (2006) *The Queen of Fats: Why Omega-3s Were Removed from the Western Diet and What We Can Do to Replace Them.* University of California Press: Berkeley, California.

Amin-Zaki, L., Ehahassani, S., Majeed, M.A., Clarkson, T.W. *et al.* (1974) 'Intra-uterine methylmercury poisoning in Iraq.' *Pediatrics*, 54: 507–595.

Amster, E., Tiwary, A. and Schenker, M.B. (2007) 'Case report: potential arsenic toxicosis secondary to herbal kelp supplement.' *Environmental Health Perspectives*, 115: 606–608.

Anderson, R.J., Bendell, D.J., Garnett, I., Groundwater, P.W. *et al.* (2002) 'Identification of indolyl-3-acryloylglycine in the urine of people with autism.' *Journal of Pharmacy and Pharmacology,* **54**: 295–298.

Aneja, A. and Tierney, E. (2008) 'Autism: the role of cholesterol in treatment.' *International Review of Psychiatry,* **20**(2): 165–170.

Antar, L.N., Afroz, R., Dictenberg, J.B., Carroll, R.C. and Bassell, G.J. (2004) 'Metabotropic glutamate receptor activation regulates Fragile X mental retardation protein and *Fmr1* mRNA localization differentially in dendrites and synapses.' *The Journal of Neuroscience,* **24**: 2648–2655.

Aschner, M., Syversen, T., Souza, D.O. and Rocha, J.B. (2006) 'Metallothioneins: mercury species-specific induction and their potential role in attenuating neurotoxicity.' *Experimental Biology and Medicine (Maywood),* **231**(9): 1468–1473.

Associate Parliamentary Food and Health Forum (2008) *The Influence of Nutrition on Mental Health: The Links Between Diet and Behaviour.* Report of an inquiry held by the Associate Parliamentary Food and Health Forum, January.

Atkins, R.C. and Herwood, R.W. (1972) *Dr. Atkins' Diet Revolution: The High Calorie Way to Stay Slim Forever.* David McKay & Co. Inc.: New York.

Atkins, R.C., Vernon, M.C. and Eberstein, J. (2004) *Atkins Diabetes Revolution: The Groundbreaking Approach to Preventing and Controlling Type 2 Diabetes.* Harper: New York.

Audette, R.V. and Gilchrist, T. (1995) *Neanderthin: A Caveman's Guide to Nutrition.* Paleolithic Press: Dallas, Texas.

Auranen, M., Vanhala, R., Varilo, T., Ayers, K. *et al.* (2002) 'A genomewide screen for autism-spectrum disorders: evidence for a major susceptibility locus on chromosome 3q25-27.' *American Journal of Human Genetics,* **71**: 777–790.

Azcarate-Peril, M.A., Bruno-Barcena, J.M., Hassan, H.M. and Klaenhammer, T.R. (2006) 'Transcriptional and functional analysis of oxalyl-coenzyme A (CoA) decarboxylase and formyl-CoA transferase genes from Lactobacillus acidophilus.' *Applied Environmental Microbiology,* **72**(3): 1891–1899.

Bakkaloglu, B., Anlar, B. Anlar, F.Y., Oktem, F. *et al.* (2008) 'Atopic features in early childhood autism.' *European Journal of Paediatric Neurology,* in press.

Banting, W. (1863) *Letter on Corpulence Addressed to the Public.* Harrison: London.

Bartzatt, R. and Beckman, J.D. (1994) 'Inhibition of phenol sulfotransferase by pyridoxal phosphate.' *Biochemistry and Pharmacology,* **47**(11): 2087–2095.

Bateman, B., Warner, J.O., Hutchinson, E., Dean, T. *et al.* (2004) 'The effects of a double blind, placebo controlled, artificial food colourings and benzoate preservative challenge on hyperactivity in a general population sample of preschool children.' *Archives of Disease in Childhood,* **89**: 506–511.

Bausell, R.B. (2007) *Snake Oil Science: The Truth About Complementary and Alternative Medicine.* Oxford University Press: Oxford.

Bear, M.F. (2005) 'Therapeutic implications of the mGluR theory of fragile X mental retardation.' *Genes, Brain and Behavior,* **4**(6): 393–398.

Bear, M.F., Huber, K.M. and Warren, S.T. (2004) 'The mGluR theory of fragile X mental retardation.' *Trends in Neurosciences,* **27**(7): 370–377.

Benga, I. (2006) 'Priorities in the discovery of the implications of water channels in epilepsy and duchenne muscular dystrophy.' *Cellular and Molecular Biology (Noisy-le-grand),* **52**(7): 46–50.

Bengmark, S. (2007) 'Advanced glycation and lipoxidation end products-amplifiers of inflammation: the role of food.' *Journal of Parenteral and Enteral Nutrition,* **31**(5): 430–440.

Bernard, C. (1865) *Introduction à l'étude de la médecine expérimentale.* Translated in 1957 by H.C. Green as *An Introduction to the Study of Experimental Medicine.* Dover: New York.

Bernstein, R.K. (2005) *The Diabetes Diet: Dr Bernstein's Low-Carbohydrate Solution.* Little, Brown & Company: New York.

Bernstein, R.K. (2007) *Dr Bernstein's Diabetes Solution: The Complete Guide to Achieving Normal Blood Sugars.* Little, Brown & Company: New York.

Best, T.H., Franz, D.N., Gilbert, D.L., Nelson, D.P. and Epstein, R.M. (2000) 'Cardiac complications in pediatric patients on the ketogenic diet.' *Neurology,* **54**(12): 2328–2330.

Bilici, M., Yildirim, F., Kandil, S., Bekaroglu, M. *et al.* (2004) 'Double-blind, placebo-controlled study of zinc sulfate in the treatment of attention deficit hyperactivity disorder.' *Progress in Neuro-Psychopharmacology & Biological Psychiatry,* **28**: 181–190.

Bilsborough, S.A. and Crowe, T.C. (2003) 'Low-carbohydrate diets: what are the potential short- and long-term health implications?' *Asia Pacific Journal of Clinical Nutrition,* **12**(4): 396–404.

Bjelakovic, G., Nikolova, D., Gluud, L.L., Simonetti, R.G. and Gluud, C. (2007) 'Mortality in randomized trials of antioxidant supplements for primary and secondary prevention systematic review and meta-analysis.' *JAMA,* **297**: 842–857.

Black, C, Kaye, J.A. and Jick, H. (2002) 'Relation of childhood gastrointestinal disorders to autism: nested case-control study using data from the UK General Practice Research Database.' *BMJ,* **325**: 419–421.

Black, J.M. (1945) 'Oxaluria in British troops in India.' *BMJ,* 28 April, 590–592.

Blaylock, R.L. (1997) *Excitotoxins: The Taste That Kills.* Health Press: Santa Fe, New Mexico.

Bodfish, J.W. (2004) 'Treating the core features of autism: are we there yet?' *Mental Retardation and Developmental Disabilities Research Reviews,* **10**(4): 318–326.

Bonamico, M., Mariani, P., Danesi, H.M., Crisogianni, M. *et al.* (2001) 'Prevalence and clinical picture of celiac disease in Italian down syndrome patients: a multicenter study.' *Journal of Pediatric Gastroenterology and Nutrition,* **33**(2): 139–143.

Bonnard, C., Durand, A., Peyrol, S., Chanseaume, E. *et al.* (2008) 'Mitochondrial dysfunction results from oxidative stress in the skeletal muscle of diet-induced insulin-resistant mice.' *The Journal of Clinical Investigation,* **118**(2): 789–800.

Boswell, J. (1799) *The Life of Samuel Johnson, LL.D.* Routledge, Warnes and Routledge: London.

Bravata, D.M., Sanders, L., Huang, J., Krumholz, H.M. *et al.* (2003) 'Efficacy and safety of low-carbohydrate diets: a systematic review.' *JAMA,* **289**(14): 1837–1850.

Brent, J., Wallace, K.L., Burkhart, K.K., Phillips, S.D. and Donovan, J.W. (eds) (2005) *Critical Care Toxicology: Diagnosis and Management of the Critically Poisoned Patient.* Elsevier Mosby: Philadelphia, Pennsylvania.

Brillat-Savarin, J.A. (1825) *'Physiologie du gout, ou Méditations de Gastronomie Transcendante; ouvrage théorique, historique et à l'ordre du jour, dédié aux Gastronomes parisiens, par un Professeur, membre de plusieurs sociétés littéraires et savantes' (The Physiology of Taste).* A. Sautelet et Cie.: Paris.

Bukelis, I., Porter, F.D., Zimmerman, A.W. and Tierney, E. (2007) 'Smith-Lemli-Opitz syndrome and autism spectrum disorder.' *American Journal of Psychiatry,* **164**(11): 1655–1661.

Burattini, M.G., Amendola, F., Aufierio, T., Spano, M. *et al.* (1990) 'Evaluation of the effectiveness of gastro-protected proteoferrin in the therapy of sideropenic anemia in childhood.' *Minerva Pediatrica,* **42**: 343–347.

Cade, R., Privette, M., Fregly, M., Rowland, N. *et al.* (2000) 'Autism and schizophrenia: intestinal disorders.' *Nutritional Neuroscience,* **3**: 57–72.

Calafat, A.M., Needham, L.L., Silva, M.J. and Lambert, G. (2004) 'Exposure to di-(2-ethylhexyl) phthalates among premature neonates in a neonatal intensive care unit.' *Pediatrics,* **113**(5): e429–434.

Cannon, G. (1987) *The Politics of Food.* Century: London.

Cannon, G. (2005) 'The rise and fall of dietetics and of nutrition science, 4000 BCE – 2000 CE.' *Public Health Nutrition,* **8**(6A): 701–705.

Casella, E.B., Valente, M., Navarro, J.M. and Kok, F. (2005) 'Vitamin B12 deficiency in infancy as a cause of developmental regression.' *Brain and Development,* **27**(8): 592–594.

Cass, H., Gringras, P., March, J., McKendrick, I. *et al.* (2008) 'Absence of urinary opioid peptides in children with autism.' *Archives of Disease in Childhood,* doi:10.1136/adc.2006.114389, published online 12 Mar 2008.

Cassady, B.A., Charboneau, N.L., Brys, E.E., Crouse, K.A., Beitz, D.C. and Wilson, T. (2007) 'Effects of low carbohydrate diets high in red meats or poultry, fish and shellfish on plasma lipids and weight loss.' *Nutrition and Metabolism,* **4**: 23. doi:10.1186/1743-7075-4-23.

Cazzullo, A.G., Musetti, M.C., Musetti, L., Bajo, S., Sacerdote, P. and Panerai, A. (1999) 'b-endorphin levels in peripheral blood mononuclear cells and long-term naltrexone treatment in autistic children.' *European Neuropsychopharmacology*, **9**(4): 361–366.

CDC (2003) *Second National Report on Human Exposure to Environmental Chemicals*. (Revised version). Centres for Disease Control and Prevention, National Center for Environmental Health: Atlanta, Georgia. NCEH Pub. No. 02-0716.

Charman, T. and Clare, P. (2004) *Mapping Autism Research: Identifying UK Priorities for the Future*. National Autistic Society: London.

Chauhan, A. and Chauhan, V. (2006) 'Oxidative stress in autism.' *Pathophysiology*, **13**: 171–181.

Chauhan, A., Chauhan, V., Brown, W.T. and Cohen, I. (2004) 'Oxidative stress in autism: increased lipid peroxidation and reduced serum levels of ceruloplasmin and transferrin – the antioxidant proteins.' *Life Sciences*, **75**: 2539–2549.

Chee, C.M., Lutchka, L., Brown, L. and Bergqvist, C. (1998) 'Ketogenic diet: unrecognized selenium deficiency.' *Epilepsia*, **39**(Suppl 6): 228 (Abstract).

Chez, M.B., Memon, S. and Hung, P.C. (2004) 'Neurologic treatment strategies in autism: an overview of medical intervention strategies.' *Seminars in Pediatric Neurology*, **11**: 229–235.

Chez, M.G., Chang, M., Krasne, V., Coughlan, C., Kominsky, M. and Schwartz, A. (2006) 'Frequency of epileptiform EEG abnormalities in a sequential screening of autistic patients with no known clinical epilepsy from 1996 to 2005.' *Epilepsy and Behavior*, **8**: 267–271.

Christison, G.W. and Ivany, K. (2006) 'Elimination diets in autism spectrum disorders: any wheat amidst the chaff?' *Journal of Developmental and Behavioral Pediatrics*, **27** (Suppl 2): S162–S171.

Ciara, E., Popowska, E., Piekutowska-Abramczuk, D., Jurkiewicz, D. *et al.* (2006) 'SLOS carrier frequency in Poland as determined by screening for Trp151X and Val326Leu DHCR7 mutations.' *European Journal of Medical Genetics*, **49**(6): 499–504.

Cleave, T.L. (1974) *The Saccharine Disease*. John Wright & Sons: Bristol. (Out of print but available from: http://journeytoforever.org/farm_library/Cleave/cleave_toc.html.)

Clements, J., Wing, L. and Dunn, G. (1986) 'Sleep problems in handicapped children: a preliminary study.' *Journal of Child Psychology and Psychiatry*, **27**(3): 399–407.

Cohen, D.J., Johnson, W.T. and Caparulo, B.K. (1976) 'Pica and elevated blood lead level in autistic and atypical children.' *American Journal of Diseases of Childhood*, **130**: 47–48.

Coleman, M. (ed.) (2005) *The Neurology of Autism*. Oxford University Press: Oxford.

Collett-Solberg, P.F. (2001) 'Diabetic ketoacidosis in children: review of pathophysiology and treatment with the use of the "two bags system".' (Article in Portuguese and English.) *Journal de Pediatrics*, **77**(1): 9–16.

Compart, P.J. and Laake, D. (2007) *The Kid-Friendly ADHD and Autism Cookbook (The Ultimate Guide to the Gluten-Free Casein-Free Diet – What It Is, Why It Works, How to Do It)*. Fair Winds Publishing: Gloucester, Maryland.

Conrad, K. (2006) *Eat Well, Feel Well: More Than 150 Delicious Specific Carbohydrate Diet (TM)-Compliant Recipes*. Clarkson Potter: New York.

Cooper, K.H. (1977) *Aerobics*. Bantam Books: New York.

Cooper, K.H. (1985) *Aerobics Program for Total Well-Being: Exercise, Diet, and Emotional Balance*. Bantam: London.

Coplan, M.J., Patch, S.C., Masters, R.D. and Bachman, M.S. (2007) 'Confirmation of and explanations for elevated blood lead and other disorders in children exposed to water disinfection and fluoridation chemicals.' *NeuroToxicology*, **28**: 1032–1042.

Cordain, L. (1999) 'Cereal grains: humanity's double-edged sword.' In: Simopoulos, A.P. (ed.) *Evolutionary Aspects of Nutrition and Health. Diet, Exercise, Genetics and Chronic Disease. World Review of Nutrition and Dietetics*, Karger: Basel, **84**: 19–73.

Cordain, L. (2002) *The Paleo Diet*. John Wiley: New York.

Cordain, L., Eaton, S.B., Miller, J.B., Mann, N. and Hill, K. (2002a) 'The paradoxical nature of hunter-gatherer diets: meat-based, yet non-atherogenic.' *European Journal of Clinical Nutrition*, **56** (Suppl 1): S42–S52.

Cordain, L., Watkins, B.A., Florant, G.L., Kelher, M., Rogers, L. and Li, Y. (2002b) 'Fatty acid analysis of wild ruminant tissues: evolutionary implications for reducing diet-related chronic disease.' *European Journal of Clinical Nutrition*, **56**: 181–191.

Cornish, E. (1998) 'A balanced approach towards healthy eating in autism.' *Journal of Human Nutrition and Dietetics*, **11**: 501–509.

Correia, C., Coutinho, A.M., Diogo, L., Grazina, M. *et al.* (2006) 'Brief report: high frequency of biochemical markers for mitochondrial dysfunction in autism: no association with the mitochondrial aspartate/glutamate carrier slc25a12 gene.' *Journal of Autism and Developmental Disorders*, **36**(8): 1137–1140.

Cory-Slechta, D.A. (2005) 'Studying toxicants as single chemicals: does this strategy adequately identify neurotoxic risk?' *NeuroToxicology*, **26**: 491–510.

Cory-Slechta, D.A., Virgolini, M.B., Thiruchelvam, M., Weston, D.D. and Bauter, M.R. (2004) 'Maternal stress modulates effects of developmental lead exposure.' *Environmental Health Perspectives*, **112**(6): 717–730.

Cory-Slechta, D.A., Virgolini, M.B., Rossi-George, A., Thiruchelvam, M., Lisek, R. and Weston, D. (2008) 'Lifetime consequences of combined maternal lead and stress.' *Basic & Clinical Pharmacology & Toxicology*, **102**: 218–227.

Croonenberghs, J., Bosmans, E., Deboutte, D., Kenis, G. and Maes, M. (2002) 'Activation of the inflammatory response system in autism.' *Neuropsychobiology*, **45**(1): 1–22.

Curhan, G.C. (1999) 'Epidemiologic evidence for the role of oxalate in idiopathic nephrolithiasis.' *Journal of Endourology*, **13**(9): 629–631.

Curhan, G.C., Willett, W.C., Speizer, F.E. and Stampfer, M.J. (1999) 'Intake of vitamins B6 and C and the risk of kidney stones in women.' *Journal of the American Society of Nephrology*, **10**(4): 840–845.

Curtin, C., Bandini, L.G., Perrin, E.C., Tybor D.J. and Must, A. (2005) 'Prevalence of overweight in children and adolescents with attention deficit hyperactivity disorder and autism spectrum disorders: a chart review.' *BMC Pediatrics*, 5: 48. doi:10.1186/1471-2431-5-48.

D'Adamo, P.J. and Whitney, C. (2002) *Eat Right for Your Type Complete Blood Type Encyclopedia*. Riverhead Books: New York.

D'Adamo, P.J. and Whitney, C. (2007) *The GenoType Diet: Change Your Genetic Destiny to Live the Longest, Fullest, and Healthiest Life Possible*. Broadway Books: New York.

D'Amelio, M., Ricci, I., Sacco, R., Liu, X. *et al.* (2005) 'Paraoxonase gene variants are associated with autism in North America, but not in Italy: possible regional specificity in gene-environment interactions.' *Molecular Psychiatry*, **10**: 1006–1016.

Dakeishi, M., Murata, K. and Grandjean, P. (2006) 'Long-term consequences of arsenic poisoning during infancy due to contaminated milk powder.' *Environmental Health: A Global Access Science Source*, available from: www.ehjournal.net/content/5/1/31.

Darwish, S.A. and Furman, B.L. (1977) 'Effects of levodopa and dopamine of plasma glucose concentration in mice.' *European Journal of Pharmacology*, 41(4): 351–360.

Das, S.K. and Ray, K. (2006) 'Wilson's disease: an update.' *Nature Clinical Practice Neurology*, **2**(9): 482–493.

de Baulny, H.O., Abadie, V., Feillet, F. and de Parscau, L. (2007) 'Management of phenylketonuria and hyperphenylalaninemia.' *Journal of Nutrition*, **137**(6)(Suppl 1): 1561S–1563S.

DeFelice, K. (2006) *Enzymes: Go with Your Gut: More Practical Guidelines for Digestive Enzymes*. Thundersnow Interactive: Johnston, Iowa.

DeFelice, K. (2008) *Enzymes for Autism and Other Neurological Conditions*. (updated 3rd edn). Thundersnow Interactive: Johnston, Iowa.

Dengate, S. (2003) *Fed Up: Understanding How Food Affects Your Child and What You Can Do About It*. Random House: Sydney, Australia.

Denke, M.A. (2001) 'Metabolic effects of high-protein, low-carbohydrate diets.' *American Journal of Cardiology*, **88**: 59–61.

De Pauw, L. and Toussaint, C. (1996) '[Primary hyperoxaluria]' [article in French]. *Revue Medicale de Bruxelles*, **17**(2): 67–74.

Devereux, G. and Seaton, A. (2005) 'Diet as a risk factor for atopy and asthma.' *Journal of Allergy and Clinical Immunology*, **115**: 1109–1117.

Diplock, A.T. (1993) 'Indexes of selenium status in human populations.' *American Journal of Clinical Nutrition Supplement*, **57**: 256S–258S.

Diplock, A.T., Charleux, J.-L., Crozier-Willi, G., Kok, F.J. *et al.* (1998) 'Functional food science and defence against reactive oxidative species.' *British Journal of Nutrition*, **80**(Suppl 1): S77–S112.

Docherty, J.P., Sack, D.A., Roffman, M., Finch, M. and Komorowski, J.R. (2005) 'A double-blind, placebo-controlled, exploratory trial of chromium picolinate in atypical depression: effect on carbohydrate craving.' *Journal of Psychiatric Practice*, **11**(5): 302–314.

Dölen, G., Osterweil, E., Rao, B.S.S., Smith, G.B. *et al.* (2007) 'Correction of fragile-X syndrome in mice.' *Neuron*, **56**(6): 955–962.

Dolinoy, D.C. Weidman, J.R. and Jirtle, R.L. (2007) 'Epigenetic gene regulation: Linking early developmental environment to adult disease.' *Reproductive Toxicology*, **23**: 297–307.

Donaldson, B.F. (1960) *Strong Medicine*. Doubleday: New York. (Also published: (1962) Cassell, London.)

Dorey, C.N. (2003) *Chemical Legacy: Contamination of the Child*. London: Greenpeace.

Duncan, S.H., Richardson, A.J., Kaul, P., Holmes, R.P., Allison, M.J. and Stewart, C.S. (2002) 'Oxalobacter formigenes and its potential role in human health.' *Applied and Environmental Microbiology*, **68**(8): 3841–3847.

Dvořáková, M., Sivonová, M., Trebatická, J., Skodáček I. *et al.* (2006) 'The effect of polyphenolic extract from pine bark, Pycnogenol on the level of glutathione in children suffering from attention deficit hyperactivity disorder (ADHD).' *Redox Reports*, **11**(4): 163–172.

Eaton, S.B. and Eaton, S.B. II (2000) 'Paleolithic vs. modern diets – selected pathophysiological implications.' *European Journal of Nutrition*, **39**: 67–70.

Editorial Board of the Atlas of Endemic Diseases and Their Environments in the People's Republic of China (1989) *The Atlas of Endemic Diseases and Their Environments in the People's Republic of China.* Science Press: Beijing, China.

Eisenberg, D., David, R.B., Ettner, S.L., Appel, S., *et al.* (1998) 'Trends in alternative medicine use in the United States, 1990–1997.' *JAMA*, **280**: 1569–1575.

Ekström, A-B., Hakenäs-Plate, L., Samuelsson, L., Tulinius, M. and Wentz, E. (2008) 'Autism spectrum conditions in myotonic dystrophy type 1: a study on 57 individuals with congenital and childhood forms.' *American Journal of Medical Genetics Part B*, doi: 10.1002/ajmg.b.30698, Epub ahead of print.

Elder, J.H., Shankar, M., Shuster, J., Theriaque, D. *et al.* (2006) 'The gluten-free, casein-free diet in autism: results of a preliminary double blind clinical trial.' *Journal of Autism and Developmental Disorders*, **36**(3): 413–420.

Ellaway, C.J., Peat, J., Williams, K., Leonard, H. and Christodoulou, J. (2001). 'Medium-term open label trial of L-carnitine in Rett syndrome.' *Brain and Development*, **23**(Suppl 1): S85–S89.

Erickson, C.A., Stigler, K.A., Corkins, M.R., Posey, D.J., Fitzgerald, J.F. and McDougle, C.J. (2005) 'Gastrointestinal factors in autistic disorder: a critical review.' *Journal of Autism and Developmental Disorders*, **35**: 713–727.

Ernsperger, L. and Stegen-Hanson, T. (2005) *Finicky Eaters: What to Do When Kids Won't Eat*. Future Horizons: Arlington, Texas.

Ernst, E. and White, A. (2000) 'The BBC survey of complementary medicine use in the UK.' *Complementary Therapies in Medicine*, **8**: 32–36.

Evangeliou, A., Vlachonikolis, I., Mihailidou, H., Spilioti, M. *et al.* (2003) 'Application of a ketogenic diet in children with autistic behavior: pilot study.' *Journal of Child Neurology*, **18**(2): 113–118.

Evans, D. (2003) *Placebo: The Belief Effect*. Harper & Collins: London.

Evans, T.A., Siedlak, S.L., Lu, L., Fu, X. *et al.* (2008) 'The autistic phenotype exhibits a remarkably localized modification of brain protein by products of free radical-induced lipid oxidation.' *American Journal of Biotechnology and Biochemistry*, **4**(2): 61–72.

Ewin, J. (2001) *Fine Wines and Fish Oil: The Life of Hugh Macdonald Sinclair*. Oxford University Press: Oxford.

Exkorn, K.S. (2005) *The Autism Sourcebook: Everything You Need to Know About Diagnosis, Coping, Treatment and Healing.* Regan Books: New York.

Fatemi, S.H., Folsom, T.D., Reutiman, T.J. and Lee, S. (2008a) 'Expression of astrocytic markers aquaporin 4 and connexin 43 is altered in brains of subjects with autism.' *Synapse,* **62**(7): 501–507.

Fatemi, S.H., Folsom, T.D., Reutiman, T.J. and Sidwell, R.W. (2008b) 'Viral regulation of aquaporin 4, connexin 43, microcephalin and nucleolin.' *Schizophrenia Research,* **98**(1–3): 163–177.

Feingold, B.F. (1975) *Why Your Child is Hyperactive.* Random House: New York.

Feingold, B.F. (1982) 'The role of diet in behaviour.' *Ecology of Disease,* **1**(2/3): 153–165.

Feingold, B.F. and Feingold, H.S. (1979) *The Feingold Cookbook for Hyperactive Children and Others with Problems Associated with Food Additives and Salicylates.* Random House: New York.

Ferguson, A.D., Labunskyy, V.M., Fomenko, D.E., Arac, D. *et al.* (2005) 'NMR structures of the selenoproteins Sep15 and SelM reveal redox activity of new thioredoxin-like family.' *Journal of Biological Chemistry,* **281**(6): 3536–3543.

Fernell, E., Fagerberg, U.L. and Hellstrom, P.M. (2007) 'No evidence for a clear link between active intestinal inflammation and autism based on analyses of faecal calprotectin and rectal nitric oxide.' *Acta Paediatrica,* **96**(7): 1076–1079.

Ferraguti, F. and Shigemoto, R. (2006) 'Metabotropic glutamate receptors.' *Cell and Tissue Research,* **326**: 483–504.

Ferrara, F., Fabietti, F., Delise, M. and Funari, E. (2005) 'Alkylphenols and alkylphenol ethoxylates contamination of crustaceans and fishes from the Adriatic Sea (Italy).' *Chemosphere,* **59**(8): 1145–1150.

Fetrow, C.H. and Avila, J.R. (2003) *Professional's Handbook of Complementary and Alternative Medicines* (3rd edn). Lippincott Williams & Wilkins: New York.

Filipek, P.A., Accardo, P.J., Baranek, G.T., Cook, E.H. Jr *et al.* (1999) 'The screening and diagnosis of autistic spectrum disorders.' *Journal of Autism and Developmental Disorders,* **29**: 437–482.

Filipek, P.A., Juranek, J., Nguyen, M.T., Cummings, C. and Gargus, J.J. (2004) 'Relative carnitine deficiency in autism.' *Journal of Autism and Developmental Disorders,* **34**(6): 615–623.

Fitzpatrick, M. (2008) *Defeating Autism: A Damaging Delusion.* Routledge: London.

Flanagan, R.J. and Jones, A.L. (2001) *Antidotes.* Taylor & Francis: London.

Fleming, R.M. (2000) 'The effect of high-protein diets on coronary blood flow.' *Angiology,* **51**(10): 817–826.

Fontcuberta, M., Arqués, J.F., Villalbí, J.R., Martínez, M. *et al.* (2008) 'Chlorinated organic pesticides in marketed food: Barcelona, 2001–06.' *Science of the Total Environment,* **389**: 52–57.

Food Standards Agency (2002) *McCance and Widdowson's The Composition of Foods* (6th edn). Royal Society of Chemistry: Cambridge.

Foster, M.W. and Sharp, R.R. (2008) 'Out of sequence: how consumer genomics could displace clinical genetics.' *Nature Review Genetics,* **9**: doi:10.1038/nrg2374.

Freedman, M.R., King, J. and Kennedy E. (2001) 'Popular diets: a scientific review.' *Obesity Research,* **9**(Suppl 1): 1S–40S.

Freeman, S.J., Roberts, W. and Daneman, D. (2005) 'Type 1 diabetes and autism.' *Diabetes Care,* **28**(4): 925–926.

Freitag, C.M. (2006) 'The genetics of autistic disorders and its clinical relevance: a review of the literature.' *Molecular Psychiatry,* **12**(1): 2–22.

Gaby, A.R. (2007) 'Natural approaches to epilepsy.' *Alternative Medicine Review,* **12**(1): 9–24.

Galli-Carminati, G., Chauvet, I. and Deriaz, N. (2006) 'Prevalence of gastrointestinal disorders in adult clients with pervasive developmental disorders.' *Journal of Intellectual Disability Research,* **50**(10): 711–718.

Gardner, C.D., Kiazand, A., Alhassan, S., Kim, S. *et al.* (2007) 'Comparison of the Atkins, Zone, Ornish, and LEARN diets for change in weight and related risk factors among overweight premenopausal women: the A to Z weight loss study: a randomized trial.' *JAMA,* **297**: 969–977.

Gardner, D.M., Shulman, K.I., Walker, S.E. and Tailor, S.A.N. (1996) 'The making of a user friendly MAOI diet.' *Journal of Clinical Psychiatry*, **57**: 99–104.

Gasior, M., Rogawski, M.A. and Hartman, A.L. (2006) 'Neuroprotective and disease-modifying effects of the ketogenic diet.' *Behavioral Pharmacology*, **17**(5–6): 431–439.

Gates, D. (2006) *The Body Ecology Diet: Recovering Your Health and Rebuilding Your Immunity* (9th edn). Body Ecology: Decatur, Georgia (available from website).

Gerlai, J. and Gerlai, R. (2003) 'Autism: a large unmet medical need and a complex research problem.' *Physiology and Behavior*, **79**: 461–470.

Gesch, C.B., Hammond, S.M., Hampson, S.E., Eves, A. and Crowder, M.J. (2002) 'Influence of supplementary vitamins, minerals and essential fatty acids on the antisocial behaviour of young adult prisoners. Randomised, placebo-controlled trial.' *British Journal of Psychiatry*, **181**: 22–28.

Ghazali, R.A. and Waring, R.H. (1999) 'The effect of flavonoids on human phenolsulphotransferases: potential in drug metabolism and chemoprevention.' *Life Sciences*, **65**(16): 1625–1632.

Giannotti, A., Tiberio, G., Castro, M., Virgilii, F. *et al.* (2001) 'Coeliac disease in Williams syndrome.' *Journal of Medical Genetics*, **38**: 767–768.

Gimeno, E., Fitó, M., Lamuela-Raventós, R.M., Castellote, A.I. *et al.* (2002) 'Effect of ingestion of virgin olive oil on human low-density lipoprotein composition.' *European Journal of Clinical Nutrition*, **56**(2): 114–120.

Gin, H., Vambergue, A., Vasseur, C., Rigalleau, V. *et al.* (2006) 'Blood ketone monitoring: a comparison between gestational diabetes and non-diabetic pregnant women.' *Diabetes and Metabolism*, **32**(6): 592–597.

Gisolfi, C.V. and Mora, F. (2000) *The Hot Brain: Survival, Temperature, and the Human Body.* MIT Press: Cambridge, Massachusetts.

Glaser, R., Kiecolt-Glaser, J.K., Marucha, P.T., MacCallum, R.C., Laskowski, B.F. and Malarkey, W.B. (1999) 'Stress-related changes in pro-inflammatory cytokine production in wounds.' *Archives of General Psychiatry*, **56**: 450–456.

Gluckman, P. and Hanson, M. (2005) *The Fetal Matrix: Evolution, Development and Disease.* Oxford University Press: Oxford.

Gluckman, P. and Hanson, M. (2006) *Mismatch: Why Our World No Longer Fits Our Bodies.* Oxford University Press: Oxford.

Godbout, R., Bergeron, C., Limoges, E., Stip, E. and Mottron, L. (2000) 'A laboratory study of sleep in Asperger's syndrome.' *Neuroreport*, **11**(1): 127–130.

Goin-Kochel, R.P., Myers, B.J. and Mackintosh, V.H. (2007) 'Parental reports on the use of treatments and therapies for children with autism spectrum disorders.' *Research in Autism Spectrum Disorders*, **11**(1): 195–209.

Goldstein, D.E., Little, R.R., Randie, R., Lorenz, R.A. *et al.* (1995) 'Tests of glycemia in diabetes.' *Diabetes Care*, **18**: 869–909.

Goodlin-Jones, B.L., Tassone, F., Gane, L.W. and Hagerman, R.J. (2004) 'Autistic spectrum disorder and the fragile X premutation.' *Journal of Developmental and Behavioral Pediatrics*, **25**: 392–398.

Gottschall, E. (1987) *Food and the Gut Reaction.* Kirkton Press: Ontario.

Gottschall, E. (1994) *Breaking the Vicious Cycle: Intestinal Health Through Diet.* Kirkton Press: Ontario.

Gottschall, E. (1997) 'Whatever happened to the cure for coeliac disease?' *Nutritional Therapy Today*, **7**(1): 8–11.

Gottschall, E. (2004) 'Digestion-gut-autism connection: the Specific Carbohydrate Diet.' *Medical Veritas*, **1**: 261–271.

Goulas, A.E., Anifantaki, K.I., Kolioulis, D.G. and Kontominas, M.G. (2000) 'Migration of di-(2-ethylhexylexyl) adipate plasticizer from food-grade polyvinyl chloride film into hard and soft cheeses.' *Journal of Dairy Science*, **83**: 1712–1718.

Grandin, T., Attwood, T., Treffert, D.A. and Rimland, B. (eds) (2006) *The Official Autism 101 Manual.* Autism Today: Seattle, Washington.

Grandjean, P. and Landrigan, P.J. (2006) 'Developmental neurotoxicity of industrial chemicals.' *The Lancet*, **368**(9553): 2167–2178.

Greenhaff, P., Gleeson, M. and Maughan, R. (1987a) 'The effect of dietary manipulation on blood acid-base status and the performance of high intensity exercise.' *European Journal of Applied Physiology*, **56**: 331–337.

Greenhaff, P., Gleeson, M. and Maughan, R. (1988) 'Diet induced metabolic acidosis and the performance of high intensity exercise in man.' *European Journal of Applied Physiology*, **57**: 583–590.

Greenhaff, P., Gleeson, M., Whiting, P. and Maughan, R. (1987b) 'Dietary composition and acid base status: limiting factors in the performance of maximal exercise in man?' *European Journal of Applied Physiology*, **56**: 444–450.

Greger, M. (2005) *Carbophobia: The Scary Truth About America's Low-Carb Craze*. Lantern Books: Herndon, Virginia.

Gromer, S., Eubel, J.M., Lee, B.L. and Jacob, J. (2005) 'Human selenoproteins at a glance.' *Cellular and Molecular Life Sciences*, **62**(21): 2414–2427.

Gu, B.Q. (1983) 'Pathology of Keshan Disease: a comprehensive review.' *Chinese Medical Journal*, **96**: 251–261.

Guenther, K., Heinke, V., Thiele, B., Kleist, E., Prast, H. and Raecker, T. (2002) 'Endocrine disrupting nonylphenols are ubiquitous in food.' *Environmental Science and Technology*, **36**(8): 1676–1680.

Haas, R.H., Rice, M.A., Trauner, D.A. and Merritt, T.A. (1986) 'Therapeutic effects of a ketogenic diet in Rett syndrome.' *American Journal of Medical Genetics*, Suppl. 1: 225–246.

Haas, S.V. (1924) 'Value of banana treatment in celiac disease.' *American Journal of Diseases of Childhood*, **28**: 421–437.

Haas, S.V. and Haas, M.P. (1951) *The Management of Celiac Disease*. J.B. Lippincott & Co.: Philadelphia, Pennsylvania.

Habgood, J. (1997) *The Hay Diet Made Easy: A Practical Guide to Food Combining with Advice on Medically Unrecognized Illness*. Souvenir Press: London.

Halsey, C.L., Collin, M.F. and Anderson, C.L. (1996) 'Extremely low-birth-weight children and their peers. A comparison of school-age outcomes.' *Archives of Pediatric and Adolescent Medicine*, **150**(8): 790–794.

Hamazaki, T., Sawazaki, S., Itomura, M., Asaoka, E. *et al.* (1996) 'The effects of docosahexaenoic acid on aggression in males.' *Journal of Clinical Investigation*, **97**: 1129–1133.

Happé, F., Ronald, A. and Plomin, R. (2006) 'Time to give up on a single explanation for autism.' *Nature: Neuroscience*, **9**: 1218–1220.

Harlan, J.R. (1992) *Crops and Man*. American Society of Agronomy: Madison, Wisconsin.

Harrington, J.W., Rosen, L., Garnecho, A. and Patrick, P.A. (2006) 'Parental perceptions and use of complementary and alternative medicine practices for children with autistic spectrum disorders in private practice.' *Journal of Developmental and Behavioral Pediatrics*, **27**: S156–S161.

Hartman, A.L., Gasior, M., Vining, E.P.G. and Rogawski, M.A. (2007) 'The neuropharmacology of the ketogenic diet.' *Pediatric Neurology*, **36**(5): 281–292.

Hebebrand, J., Henninghausen, K., Nau, S., Himmelmann, G.W. *et al.* (1997) 'Low body weight in male children and adolescents with schizoid personality disorder or Asperger's disorder.' *Acta Psychiatrica Scandinavica*, **96**(1):64–67.

Hediger, M.L., England, L.J., Molloy, C.A., Yu, K.F., Manning-Courtney, P. and Mills, J.L. (2007) 'Reduced bone cortical thickness in boys with autism or autism spectrum disorder.' *Journal of Autism and Developmental Disorders* [Epub ahead of print], doi: 10.1007/s10803-007-0453-6.

Heller, R.F. and Heller, R.F. (1997) *Carbohydrate-Addicted Kids: Help Your Child or Teen Break Free of Junk Food and Sugar Cravings – For Life!* HarperCollins: New York.

Hendler, S.S. and Rorvik, D. (eds) (2001) *PDR for Nutritional Supplements*. Thompson PDR: Montvale, New Jersey.

Herbert, J.D., Sharp, I.R. and Gaudiano, B.A. (2002) 'Separating fact from fiction in the etiology and treatment of autism: a scientific review of the evidence.' *The Scientific Review of Mental Health Practice*, **1**(1): 23–43.

Herrick, K., Phillips, D.I.W., Haselden, S., Shiell, A.W., Campbell-Brown, M. and Godfrey, K.M. (2003) 'Maternal consumption of a high-meat, low-carbohydrate diet in late pregnancy: relation to adult cortisol concentrations in the offspring.' *The Journal of Clinical Endocrinology and Metabolism*, **88**(8): 3554–3560.

Hess, B., Jost, C., Zipperle, L., Takkinen, R. and Jaeger, P. (1998) 'High-calcium intake abolishes hyperoxaluria and reduces urinary crystallization during a 20-fold normal oxalate load in humans.' *Nephrology, Dialysis and Transplantation*, **13**: 2241–2247.

Heyman, M.B. (2006) 'Lactose intolerance in infants, children, and adolescents.' *Pediatrics*, **118**(3): 1279–1286.

Hibuse, T., Maeda, N., Funahashi, T., Yamamoto, K. *et al.* (2005) 'Aquaporin 7 deficiency is associated with development of obesity through activation of adipose glycerol kinase.' *PNAS*, **102**(31): 10993–10998.

Hicks, M., Ferguson, S., Bernier, F. and Lemay, J.-F. (2008) 'A case report of monozygotic twins with Smith-Magenis syndrome.' *Journal of Developmental and Behavioural Pediatrics*, **29**: 42–46.

Hiilamo, H.T. (2007) 'The impact of strategic funding by the tobacco industry of medical expert witnesses appearing for the defence in the Aho Finnish product liability case.' *Addiction*, **102**: 979–988.

Ho, K.J., Mikkelson, B., Lewis, L.A., Feldman, S.A. and Taylor, C.B. (1972) 'Alaskan Arctic Eskimos: responses to a customary high fat diet.' *American Journal of Clinical Nutrition*, **25**: 737–745.

Hodson, A.H. (1992) 'Empirical use of exclusion diets in chronic disorders: discussion paper.' *Journal of the Royal Society of Medicine*, **85**: 556–559.

Holford, P. and Colson, D. (2006) *Optimum Nutrition for Your Child's Mind: Maximize Your Child's Potential.* Piatkus: London.

Hollander, E. and Anagnostou, E. (2007) *Clinical Manual for the Treatment of Autism.* American Psychiatric Publishing Inc.: Arlington, Virginia.

Holmes, A.S., Blaxill, M.F. and Haley, B.E. (2003) 'Reduced levels of mercury in first baby haircuts of autistic children.' *International Journal of Toxicology*, **22**: 277–285.

Holtmeier, W. and Caspary, W.F. (2006) 'Celiac disease.' *Orphanet Journal of Rare Diseases*, **1**: 3, doi:10.1186/1750-1172-1-3.

Horrobin, D. (2001) *The Madness of Adam and Eve: How Schizophrenia Shaped Humanity.* Random House: London.

Horvath, K., Medeiros, L. and Rabszlyn, A. (2000) 'High prevalence of gastrointestinal symptoms in autistic children with autistic spectrum disorder.' *Journal of Pediatric Gastroenterology and Nutrition*, **31**: S174.

Horvath, K., Papadimitriou, J.C., Rabsztyn, A., Drachenberg, C. and Tildon, J.T. (1999) 'Gastrointestinal abnormalities in children with autistic disorder.' *Journal of Pediatrics*, **135**: 559–563.

Horvath, K. and Perman, J.A. (2002a) 'Autism and gastrointestinal symptoms.' *Current Gastroenterology Reports*, **4**: 251–258.

Horvath, K. and Perman, J.A. (2002b) 'Autistic disorder and gastrointestinal disease.' *Current Opinion in Pediatrics*, **14**: 583–587.

Hougaard, K.S. and Hansen, A.M. (2007) 'Enhancement of developmental toxicity effects of chemicals by gestational stress. A review.' *Neurotoxicology and Teratology*, **29**: 425–445.

Houlihan, J., Wiles, R., Thayer, K. and Gray, S. (2003) *Body Burden. The Pollution in People.* Washington, DC, USA: Environmental Working Group.

Howell, M. and Ford, P. (1985) *The Ghost Disease and Twelve Other Stories of Detective Work in the Medical Field.* Penguin Books: Harmondsworth.

Howlin, P. (1998) 'Practitioner review: psychological and educational treatments for autism.' *Journal of Child Psychology and Psychiatry*, **39**(3): 307–322.

Hoyt, C.S. III and Billson, F.A. (1977) 'Low-carbohydrate diet optic neuropathy.' *Medical Journal of Australia*, **1**: 65–66.

Hunter, L.C., O'Hare, A., Herron, W.J., Fisher, L.A. and Jones, G.E. (2003) 'Opioid peptides and dipeptidyl peptidase in autism.' *Developmental Medicine and Child Neurology*, **45**: 121–128.

Isbister, G.K. and Kiernan, M.C. (2005) 'Neurotoxic marine poisoning.' *Lancet: Neurology,* **4**: 219–228.

Izaka, K.I., Yamada, M., Kawano, T. and Suyama, T. (1972) 'Gastrointestinal absorption and antiinflammatory effect of bromelain.' *Japanese Journal of Pharmacology,* **22**(4): 519–534.

Jaeger, R.J. and Rubin, R.J. (1973) 'Extraction, localization and metabolism of di-2-ethylhexyl phthalate from PVC medical devices.' *Environmental Health Perspectives,* **3**: 95–102.

Jamain, S., Betancur, C., Quach, H., Philippe, A. *et al.* (2002) 'Linkage and association of the glutamate receptor 6 gene with autism.' *Molecular Psychiatry,* **7**(3): 302–310.

James, S.J., Cutler, P., Melnyk, S., Jernigan, S. *et al.* (2004) 'Metabolic biomarkers of increased oxidative stress and impaired methylation capacity in children with autism.' *American Journal of Clinical Nutrition,* **80**(6): 1611–1617.

Jepson, B., Wright, K. and Johnson, J. (2007) *Changing the Course of Autism: A Scientific Approach for Parents and Physicians.* Sentient Publications: Boulder, Colorado.

Jesner, O.S., Aref-Adib, M. and Coren, E. (2007) 'Risperidone for autism spectrum disorder (Review).' *Cochrane Database of Systematic Reviews,* Issue **1**, Art. No.: CD005040. DOI: 10.1002/14651858.CD005040.pub2.

Jimenez, E.C., Donevan, S., Walker, C., Zhou, L.M. *et al.* (2002) 'Conantokin-L, a new NMDA receptor antagonist: determinants for anticonvulsant potency.' *Epilepsy Research,* **51**(1–2): 73–80.

Jones, M. (2007) *Feast: Why Humans Share Food.* Oxford University Press: Oxford.

Jones, A.W. and Rossner, S. (2007) 'False-positive breath-alcohol test after a ketogenic diet.' *International Journal of Obesity,* **31**: 559–561.

Junien, C. (2006) 'Impact of diets and nutrients/drugs on early epigenetic programming.' *Journal of Inherited Metabolic Disease,* **29**: 359–365.

Kadereit, B., Kumar, P., Wang, W.-J., Miranda, D. *et al.* (2008) 'Evolutionarily conserved gene family important for fat storage.' *PNAS,* **105**(1): 94–99.

Kang, H.-C., Lee, Y.-M., Kim, H.D., Lee, J.S. and Slama, A. (2007) 'Safe and effective use of the ketogenic diet in children with epilepsy and mitochondrial respiratory chain complex defects.' *Epilepsia,* **48**(1): 82–88.

Kaplan, B.J. and Shannon, S. (2007) 'Nutritional aspects of child and adolescent psychopharmacology.' *Pediatric Annals,* **36**(9): 600–609.

Katahn, M. (1987) *The Rotation Diet.* Bantam: New York.

Kauffman, J.M. (2004) 'Low-carbohydrate diets.' *Journal of Scientific Exploration,* **18**(1): 83–134.

Kellow, J., Costain, L. and Walton, R. (2008) *The Calorie, Carb and Fat Bible 2008.* Weight Loss Resources Ltd.: Peterborough.

Kemper, M.J., Conrad, S. and Muller-Wiefel, D.E. (1997) 'Primary hyperoxaluria type 2.' *European Journal of Pediatrics,* **156**: 509–512.

Kenton, L. (2002) *The X Factor Diet: For Lasting Weight Loss and Vital Health.* Vermillion: London.

Keshan Disease Research Group (1979) 'Epidemiologic studies on the etiologic relationship of selenium and Keshan disease.' *Chinese Medical Journal,* **92**: 477–482.

Keys, A. (1959) *Eat Well and Stay Well.* DoubleDay: New York.

Keys, A. and Keys, M. (1975) *How to Eat Well and Stay Well the Mediterranean Way.* DoubleDay: New York.

Kidd, P.M. (2002) 'Autism, an extreme challenge to integrative medicine. Part II: medical management.' *Alternative Medicine Review,* **7**(6): 472–499.

Kim, W., Erlandsen, H., Surendran, S., Stevens, R.C. *et al.* (2004) 'Trends in enzyme therapy for phenylketonuria.' *Molecular Therapy,* **10**: 220–224.

Klavdieva, M.M. (1996) 'The history of neuropeptides IV.' *Frontiers in Neuroendocrinology,* **17**: 247–280.

Klein, A.J., Armstrong, B.L., Greer, M.K. and Brown, F.R. 3rd (1990) 'Hyperacusis and otitis media in individuals with Williams syndrome.' *Journal of Speech and Hearing Disorders,* **55**(2): 339–344.

Klepper, J., Diefenbach, S., Kohlschutter, A. and Voit, T. (2004) 'Effects of the ketogenic diet in the glucose transporter 1 deficiency syndrome.' *Prostaglandins, Leukotrienes and Essential Fatty Acids*, **70**: 321–327.

Klepper, J. and Leiendecker, B. (2007) 'GLUT1 deficiency syndrome – 2007 update.' *Developmental Medicine and Child Neurology*, **49**(9): 707–716.

Knapp, M., Romeo, R. and Beecham, J. (2008) *The Economic Consequences of Autism in the UK*. Foundation for People with Learning Disabilities: London.

Knivsberg, A.M., Reichelt, K.L., Hoien, T. and Nodland, M. (2002) 'A randomised, controlled study of dietary intervention in autistic syndromes.' *Nutritional Neuroscience*, **5**(4): 251–261.

Knivsberg, A.M., Reichelt, K.L. and Nodland, M. (2000) 'Reports on dietary intervention in autistic disorders.' *Nutritional Neuroscience*, **4**: 25–37.

Kondo, K. (2000) 'Congenital Minamata disease: warnings from Japan's experience.' *Journal of Child Neurology*, **15**: 458–464.

Kossoff, E.H. (2004) 'More fat and fewer seizures: dietary therapies for epilepsy.' *Lancet: Neurology*, **3**: 415–420.

Kossoff, E.H., Krauss, G.L., McGrogan, J.R. and Freeman, J.M. (2003) 'Efficacy of the Atkins diet as therapy for intractable epilepsy.' *Neurology*, **61**: 1789–1791.

Kossoff, E.H., Turner, Z., Bluml, R.M., Pyzik, P.L., Eileen, P.G. and Vining, E.P.G. (2007) 'A randomized, crossover comparison of daily carbohydrate limits using the modified Atkins diet.' *Epilepsy and Behavior*, **10**: 432–436.

Kozielec, T. and Starobrat-Hermelin, B. (1997) 'Assessment of magnesium levels in children with ADHD.' *Magnesium Research*, **10**: 143–148.

Krummel, D.A., Seligson, F.H. and Guthrie, H.A. (1996) 'Hyperactivity: is candy causal?' *Critical Reviews in Food Science and Nutrition*, **36**(1–2): 31–47.

Kulman, G., Lissini, P., Rovelli, F., Roselli, M.S., Brivio, F. and Sequeri, P. (2000) 'Evidence of pineal endocrine hypofunction in autistic children.' *Neuroendocrinology Letters*, **21**: 31–34.

Kurtz, L.A. (2008) *Understanding Controversial Therapies for Children with Autism, Attention Deficit Disorder and Other Learning Disabilities*. Jessica Kingsley Publishers: London.

Laidlaw, S.A., Shultz, T.D., Cecchino, J.T. and Kopple, J.D. (1988) 'Plasma and urine taurine levels in vegans.' *American Journal of Clinical Nutrition*, **47**: 660–663.

Lang, T. (2003) 'Food industrialization and food power: implications for food governance.' *Development Policy Review*, **21**(5): 555–568.

Lau, K., McLean, W.G., Williams, D.P. and Howard, C.V. (2006) 'Synergistic interactions between commonly used food additives in a developmental neurotoxicity test.' *Toxicological Sciences*, **90**(1): 178–187.

Learning and Developmental Disabilities Initiative (2008) *Scientific Consensus Statement on Environmental Agents Associated with Neurodevelopmental Disorders*. Consensus Statement, 20 February, available from www.iceh.org/pdfs/LDDI/LDDIStatement.pdf.

Lee, L., Turner, L., Goldberg, B. and Leviton, R. (1998) *The Enzyme Cure: How Plant Enzymes Can Help You Relieve 36 Health Problems*. Prentice Hall: Upper Saddle River, New Jersey.

Legge, B. (2002) *Can't Eat, Won't Eat: Dietary Difficulties and Autistic Spectrum Disorders*. Jessica Kingsley Publishers: London.

Lemann, J. Jr, Pleuss, J.A., Worcester, E.M., Hornick, L., Schrab, D. and Hoffmann, R.G. (1996) 'Urinary oxalate excretion increases with body size and decreases with increasing dietary calcium intake among healthy adults.' *Kidney International*, **49**: 200–208.

Levine, M., Conry-Cantilena, C., Wang, Y., Welch, R.W. *et al.* (1996) 'Vitamin C pharmacokinetics in healthy volunteers: evidence for a recommended dietary allowance (ascorbic acid/bioavailability).' *Proceedings of the National Academy of Science USA*, **93**: 3704–3709.

Levy, S.E. and Hyman, S.L. (2005) 'Novel treatments for autistic spectrum disorders.' *Mental Retardation and Developmental Disabilities Research Reviews*, **11**: 131–142.

Levy, S.E., Mandell, D.S., Merhar, S., Ittenbach, R.F. and Pinto-Martin, J.A. (2003) 'Use of complementary and alternative medicine among children recently diagnosed with autistic spectrum disorder.' *Journal of Developmental and Behavioral Pediatrics*, **24**(6): 418–423.

Levy, S.E., Souders, M.C., Ittenbach, R.F., Giarelli, E., Mulberg, A.E. and Pinto-Martin, J.A. (2007) 'Relationship of dietary intake to gastrointestinal symptoms in children with autistic spectrum disorders.' *Biological Psychiatry*, **61**: 492–497.

Lewis, L. (1999) *Special Diets for Special Kids: Understanding and Implementing Special Diets to Aid in the Treatment of Autism and Related Developmental Disorders.* Jessica Kingsley Publishers: London.

Lieb, C.W. (1929) 'The effects on human beings of a twelve months' exclusive meat diet.' *Journal of the American Medical Association*, **93**:20–22.

Liebman, M. and Costa, G. (2000) 'Effects of calcium and magnesium on urinary oxalate excretion after oxalate loads.' *Journal of Urology*, **163**: 1565–1569.

Liepins, R. and Pearce, E.M. (1976) 'Chemistry and toxicity of flame retardants for plastics.' *Environmental Health Perspectives*, **17**: 55–63.

Lightdale, J.R., Siegel, B. and Heyman, M.B. (2001) 'Gastrointestinal symptoms in autistic children.' *Clinical Perspectives on Gastroenterology*, **1**: 56–58.

Lilienfeld, S.O. (2005) 'Scientifically unsupported and supported interventions for childhood psychopathology: a summary.' *Pediatrics*, **115**: 761–764.

Lindstrom, M. and Seybold, P.B. (2004) *Brand Child: Remarkable Insights into the Minds of Today's Global Kids and Their Relationships with Brands (revised edn).* Kogan Page: London.

Lininger, S.W., Gaby, A.R., Austin, S., Batz, F. *et al.* (1999) *The A–Z Guide to Drug-Herb-Vitamin Interactions.* Prima Publishing: New York.

Lipski, E. (2004) *Digestive Wellness.* McGraw Hill: New York.

Lipski, E. (2006) *Digestive Wellness for Children: How to Strengthen the Immune System and Prevent Disease Through Healthy Digestion.* Basic Health Publications: Laguna Beach, California.

Lissoni, G., Rovelli, P., Roselli, M.G., Brivio, F. and Sequeri, P. (2002) 'Evidence of pineal endocrine hypofunction in autistic children.' *Neurology and Endocrinology Letters*, **21**(1): 31–34.

Luban, R., Reis-Bahrami, K. and Shoert, B. (2006) 'I want to say one word to you – just one word – "plastics".' *Transfusion*, **46**(4): 503–506.

Luscombe-Marsh, N.D., Noakes, M., Wittert, G.A., Keogh, J.B., Foster, P. and Clifton, P.M. (2005) 'Carbohydrate-restricted diets high in either monounsaturated fat or protein are equally effective at promoting fat loss and improving blood lipids.' *American Journal of Clinical Nutrition*, **81**: 762–772.

Luyt, D., Dunbar, H. and Baker, H. (2000) 'Nut allergy in children: investigation and management.' *Journal of the Royal Society of Medicine*, **93**(6): 283–287.

McCandless, J. (2007) *Children with Starving Brains: A Medical Treatment Guide for Autism Spectrum Disorder* (3rd edn). Bramble Books: Putney, Vermont.

McCann, D., Barrett, A., Cooper, A., Crumpler, D. *et al.* (2007) 'Food additives and hyperactive behaviour in 3-year-old and 8/9-year-old children in the community: a randomised, double-blinded, placebo-controlled trial.' *Lancet*, **370**(9598): 1560–1567.

McCarthy, J. (2007) *Louder Than Words: A Mother's Journey in Healing Autism.* Dutton Adult (Penguin USA): New York.

Macdonald, A., Daly, A., Davies, P., Asplin, D. *et al.* (2004) 'Protein substitutes for PKU: what's new?' *Journal of Inherited Metabolic Disease*, **27**: 363–371.

McDougle, C.J., Naylor, S.T., Cohen, D.J., Aghajanian, G.K., Heninger, G.R. and Price, L.H. (1996) 'Effects of tryptophan depletion in drug-free adults with autistic disorder.' *Archives of General Psychiatry*, **53**(11): 993–1000.

McFadden, S.A. (1996) 'Phenotypic variation in xenobiotic metabolism and adverse environmental response: focus on sulfur-dependent detoxification pathways.' *Toxicology*, **III**(1–3): 43–65.

Mackarness, R. (1958) *Eat Fat and Grow Slim.* Harvill Press: London. (Revised and extended edition: 1975 (Fontana/Collins: London).)

Mackarness, R. (1959) 'Stone age diet for functional disorders.' *Medical World*, **91**: 14–19.

Mackarness, R. (1976) *Not All in the Mind.* Pan: London.

Mackarness, R. (1980) *Chemical Victims.* Pan: London.

MacLennan, A.H., Wilson, D.H. and Taylor, A.W. (1996) 'Prevalence and cost of alternative medicine in Australia.' *Lancet,* **347**(9001): 569–573.

Mamoulakis, D., Galanakis, E., Dionyssopoulou, E., Evangeliou, A. and Sbyrakis, S. (2004) 'Carnitine deficiency in children and adolescents with type 1 diabetes.' *Journal of Diabetes Complications,* **18**(5): 271–274.

Mann, K.K., Davison, K., Colombo, M., Colosimo, A.L. *et al.* (2006) 'Antimony trioxide-induced apoptosis is dependent on SEK1/JNK signaling.' *Toxicology Letters,* **160**: 158–170.

Mann, N. (2000) 'Dietary lean red meat and human evolution.' *European Journal of Nutrition,* **39**: 71–79.

Marohn, S. (2002) *The Natural Medicine Guide to Autism.* Hampton Roads Publishing: Charlottesville, Virginia.

Massey, L.K. and Smith, R.L. (1993) 'Effect of dietary oxalate and calcium on urinary oxalate and risk of formation of calcium oxalate kidney stones.' *Journal of the American Dietetic Association,* **93**: 901.

Masters, R.D. and Coplan, M.J. (1999) 'Water treatment with silicofluorides and lead toxicity.' *International Journal of Environmental Studies,* **56**: 435–449.

Matalon, R., Michals-Matalon, K., Bhatia, G., Burlina, A.B. *et al.* (2007) 'Double blind placebo control trial of large neutral amino acids in treatment of PKU: effect on blood phenylalanine.' *Journal of Inherited Metabolic Disease,* **30**(2): 153–158.

Megson, M. (2000) 'Is autism a G-alpha protein defect reversible with natural vitamin A?' *Medical Hypotheses,* **54**(6): 979–983.

Meharg, A.A. (2005) *Venomous Earth: How Arsenic Caused the World's Worst Mass Poisoning.* Macmillan: Basingstoke.

Melke, J., Goubran-Botros, H., Chaste, P., Betancur, C. *et al.* and the PARIS study (2008) 'Abnormal melatonin synthesis in autism spectrum disorders.' *Molecular Psychiatry,* **13**(1): 90–98.

Melmed, R.D., Schneider, C.K., Fabes, R.A., Phillips, J. and Reichelt, K. (2000) 'Metabolic markers and gastrointestinal symptoms in children with autism and related disorders.' *Journal of Pediatric Gastroenterology and Nutrition,* **3**: S31–S32.

Mendelsohn, N.J. and Schaefer, G.B. (2008) 'Genetic evaluation of autism.' *Seminars in Pediatric Neurology,* **15**: 27–31.

Menon, M. and Mahle, C.J. (1982) 'Oxalate metabolism and renal calculi.' *Journal of Urology,* **127**: 148–151.

Michelson, A.M. (1998) 'Selenium glutathione peroxidase: some aspects in man.' *Journal of Environmental Pathology Toxicology and Oncology,* **17**(3–4): 233–239.

Millichap, J.G. and Yee, M. (2003) 'The diet factor in pediatric and adolescent migraine.' *Pediatric Neurology,* **28**: 9–15.

Millward, C., Ferriter, M., Calver, S. and Connell-Jones, G. (2008) 'Gluten- and casein-free diets for autistic spectrum disorder.' *Cochrane Database Systematic Reviews,* **2**: CD003498.

Milton, K. (2000) 'Hunter-gatherer diets – a different perspective.' *American Journal of Clinical Nutrition,* **71**: 665–667.

Moynahan, B. (1998) *Rasputin: The Saint who Sinned.* Aurum Press: London.

MRC (2001) *MRC Review of Autism Research: Epidemiology and Causes.* Medical Research Council: London (www.mrc.ac.uk).

Muehlmann, A.M. and Devine, D.P. (2008) 'Glutamate-mediated neuroplasticity in an animal model of self-injurious behaviour.' *Behavioural Brain Research,* **189**(1): 32–40.

Mullenix, P.J., Denbesten, P.K., Schunior, A. and Kernan, W.J. (1995) 'Neurotoxicity of sodium fluoride in rats.' *Neurotoxicology and Teratology,* **17**(2): 169–177.

Murch, S. (2003) 'Separating speculation from inflammation in autism.' *The Lancet,* **362**(9394): 1498–1499.

Murphy, E.A. and Aucott, M. (1999) 'A methodology to assess the amounts of pesticidal mercury used historically in New Jersey.' *Soil and Sediment Contamination,* **8**(1): 131–148.

Nataf, R., Skorupka, C., Amet, L., Lam, A., Springbett, A. and Lathe, R. (2006) 'Porphyrinuria in childhood autistic disorder: implications for environmental toxicity.' *Toxicology and Applied Pharmacology*, **214**(2): 99–108.

Neal, E.G., Chaffe, H., Schwartz, R.H., Lawson, M.S. *et al.* (2008) 'The ketogenic diet for the treatment of childhood epilepsy: a randomised controlled trial.' *Lancet: Neurology*, Published online 3 May 2008, DOI: 10.1016/S1474-4422(08)70092-9.

Needleman, H. (2004) 'Lead poisoning.' *Annual Review of Medicine*, **55**: 209–222.

Nesse, R.M. and Williams, G.C. (1994) *Evolution and Healing: The New Science of Darwinian Medicine.* Random House: New York.

Neve, J. (1996) 'Selenium as a risk factor for cardiovascular diseases.' *Journal of Cardiovascular Risk*, **3**: 42–47.

Noble, D. (2006) *The Music of Life: Biology Beyond the Genome.* Oxford University Press: Oxford.

Nordli, D. (2002) 'The ketogenic diet: uses and abuses.' *Neurology*, **58**: 21–24.

Novelli, G. and Reichardt, J.K.V. (2000) 'Molecular basis of disorders of human galactose metabolism: past, present, and future.' *Molecular Genetics and Metabolism*, **71**: 62–65.

Oades, R.D., Daniels, R. and Rascher, W. (1998) 'Plasma neuropeptide-Y levels, monoamine metabolism, electrolyte excretion and drinking behavior in children with attention-deficit hyperactivity disorder.' *Psychiatry Research*, **80**(2): 177–186.

Obeid, R. and Herrmann, W. (2006) 'Priorities in the discovery of the implications of water channels in epilepsy and Duchenne muscular dystrophy.' *Cellular and Molecular Biology (Noisy-le-grand)*, **52**(5): 16–20.

Ohira, M. and Aoyama, H. (1973) 'Epidemiological studies on the Morinaga powdered milk poisoning incident [in Japanese].' *Nippon Eiseigaku Zasshi*, **27**: 500–531.

Okafor, P.N. (2004) 'Assessment of cyanide overload in cassava consuming populations of Nigeria and the cyanide content of some cassava based foods.' *African Journal of Biotechnology*, **3**(7): 358–361.

Oliveira, G., Ataíde, A., Marques, C., Miguel, T.S. *et al.* (2007) 'Epidemiology of autism spectrum disorder in Portugal: prevalence, clinical characterization, and medical conditions.' *Developmental Medicine and Child Neurology*, **49**: 726–733.

Oliveira, G., Diogo, L., Grazina, M., Garcia, P. *et al.* (2005) 'Mitochondrial dysfunction in autism spectrum disorders: a population-based study.' *Developmental Medicine and Child Neurology*, **47**: 185–189.

Olson, M.J., Handler, J.A. and Thurman, R.G. (1986) 'Mechanism of zone-specific hepatic steatosis caused by valproate: inhibition of ketogenesis in periportal regions of the liver lobule.' *Molecular Pharmacology*, **30**(6): 520–525.

Osuntokun, B.O., Monekosso, G.L. and Wilson, J. (1969) 'Relationship of a degenerative tropical neuropathy to diet: report of a field survey.' *British Medical Journal*, **1**: 547–550.

Oyane, N.M. and Bjorvatn, B. (2005) 'Sleep disturbances in adolescents and young adults with autism and Asperger syndrome.' *Autism*, **9**(1): 83–94.

Pain, S. (2008) 'Marvellous mithridatium.' *New Scientist*, **197**(2640): 52–53.

Pangborn, J. and Baker, S.M. (2005) *Autism: Effective Biomedical Treatments.* Autism Research Institute: San Diego, California.

Panksepp, J. (1979) 'A neurochemical theory of autism.' *Trends in the Neurosciences*, **2**: 174–177.

Papas, A.M. (ed.) (1999) *Antioxidant Status, Diet, Nutrition and Health.* CRC Press: Boca Raton, Florida.

Pardo, C.A. and Eberhart, C.G. (2007) 'The neurobiology of autism.' *Brain Pathology*, **17**: 434–447.

Pedersen, H. and Hartmann, J. (2004) *Toxic Childrenswear by Disney: Worldwide Investigation of Hazardous Chemicals in Disney Clothes.* Greenpeace: Brussels.

Pennington, A.W. (1953a) 'An alternate approach to obesity.' *American Journal of Clinical Nutrition*, **1**(2): 100–106.

Pennington, A.W. (1953b) 'Treatment of obesity with calorie unrestricted diets.' *American Journal of Clinical Nutrition*, **1**(5): 343–348.

Peräaho, M., Collin, P., Kaukinen, K., Kekkonen, L., Miettinen, S. and Mäki, M. (2004a) 'Oats can diversify a gluten-free diet in celiac disease and dermatitis herpetiformis.' *Journal of the American Dietetic Association*, **104**(7): 1148–1150.

Peräaho, M., Kaukinen, K., Mustalahti, K., Vuolteenaho, N. *et al.* (2004b) 'Effect of an oats-containing gluten-free diet on symptoms and quality of life in coeliac disease. A randomized study.' *Scandinavian Journal of Gastroenterology*, **39**(1): 27–31.

Peregrin, T. (2007) 'Registered dietitians' insights in treating autistic children.' *Journal of the American Dietetic Association*, **107**(5): 727–730.

Peters, L.D., Doyotte, A., Mitchelmore, C.L., McEvoy, J. and Livingstone, D.R. (2001) 'Seasonal variation and estradiol-dependent elevation of Thames estuary eel Anguilla anguilla plasma vitellogenin levels and comparisons with other United Kingdom estuaries.' *Science of the Total Environment*, **279**(1–3): 137–150.

Peters, R.J.B. (2005) 'Chemical Additives in Consumer Products.' Available from: http://www.greenpeace.org/international/press/reports/chemical-additives-in-consumer

Pliszka, S.R. (2003) *Neuroscience for the Mental Health Clinician*. Guildford Press: New York.

Plotkin, M.J. (2000) *Medicine Quest: In Search of Nature's Healing Secrets*. Viking Press (Penguin): New York.

Poling, J.S., Frye, R.E., Shoffner, J. and Zimmerman, A.W. (2006) 'Developmental regression and mitochondrial dysfunction in a child with autism.' *Journal of Child Neurology*, **21**(2): 170–172.

Posey, D.J., Erickson, C.A., Stigler, K.A. and McDougle, C.J. (2006) 'The use of selective serotonin reuptake inhibitors in autism and related disorders.' *Journal of Child and Adolescent Psychopharmacology*, **16**(1–2): 181–186.

Potocki, L., Bi, W., Treadwell-Deering, D., Carvalho, C.M. *et al.* (2007) 'Characterization of Potocki-Lupski syndrome (dup(17)(p11.2p11.2)) and delineation of a dosage-sensitive critical interval that can convey an autism phenotype.' *American Journal of Human Genetics*, **80**(4): 633–649.

Poustie, V.J., Wildgoose, J. and Rutherford, P. (1999) 'Dietary interventions for phenylketonuria.' *Cochrane Database of Systematic Reviews*, Issue 3. Art. No.: CD001304. DOI: 10.1002/14651858.CD001304.

Prasad, R. (2008) *Recipes for the Specific Carbohydrate Diet: The Grain-Free, Lactose-Free, Sugar-Free Solution to IBD, Celiac Disease, Autism, Cystic Fibrosis, and Other Health Conditions*. Fair Winds Press: Beverley, Massachusetts.

Pratt, C.H. (1928) 'The treatment of epilepsy.' *Canadian Medical Association Journal*, **19**(3): 303–312.

Purcell, A.E., Jeon, O.H., Zimmerman, A.W., Blue, M.E. and Pevsner, J. (2001) 'Postmortem brain abnormalities of the glutamate neurotransmitter system in autism.' *Neurology*, **57**(9): 1618–1628.

Rajasekar, P. and Anuradha, C.V. (2007) 'Effect of L-carnitine on skeletal muscle lipids and oxidative stress in rats fed high-fructose diet.' *Experimental Diabetes Research*, **2007**, Article ID 72741, 8 pages, doi:10.1155/2007/72741.

Ramoz, N., Reichert, J.G., Smith, C.J., Silverman, J.M. *et al.* (2004) 'Linkage and association of the mitochondrial aspartate/glutamate carrier SLC25A12 gene with autism.' *American Journal of Psychiatry*, **161**(4): 662–669.

Rana, S.K. and Sanders, T.A.B. (1986) 'Taurine concentrations in the diet, plasma, urine and breast milk of vegans compared with omnivores.' *British Journal of Nutrition*, **56**: 17–27.

Raszeja-Wyszomirska, J., Kurzawski, G., Suchy, J., Zawada, I., Jan Lubinski, J. and Milkiewicz, P. (2008) 'Frequency of mutations related to hereditary haemochromatosis in northwestern Poland.' *Journal of Applied Genetics*, **49**(1): 105–107.

Ratnesar, S. (2002) *The Omega-3 Life Program: Your Food Guide for Health and Healing*. McGraw-Hill Australia: Sydney.

Reichelt, K.L. and Knivsberg, A.M. (2003) 'Can the pathophysiology of autism be explained by the nature of the discovered urine peptides?' *Nutritional Neuroscience*, **6**: 19–28.

Richardson, A. (2006a) *They Are What You Feed Them: How Food Can Improve Your Child's Behaviour, Learning and Mood*. Harper Thorsons: London.

Richardson, A.J. (2006b) 'Omega-3 fatty acids in ADHD and related neurodevelopmental disorders.' *International Review of Psychiatry*, **18**(2): 155–172.

Richdale, A.L. and Prior, M.R. (1995) 'The sleep/wake rhythm in children with autism.' *European Child and Adolescent Psychiatry*, **4**(3): 175–186.

Ring, H., Woodbury-Smith, M., Watson, P., Wheelwright, S. and Baron-Cohen, S. (2008) 'Clinical heterogeneity among people with high functioning autism spectrum conditions: evidence favouring a continuous severity gradient.' *Behavioral and Brain Functions*, **4**: 11, doi:10.1186/1744-9081-4-11.

Robinson, J. (2004) *Pasture Perfect: The Far-Reaching Benefits of Choosing Meat, Eggs, and Dairy Products from Grass-Fed Animals*. Vashon Island Press: Vashon, Washington.

Robison, J.E. (2007) *Look Me in the Eye: My Life with Asperger's*. Random House, Ebury Press: London.

Rodriguez, J.C. (2007) *The Diet Selector: From Atkins to the Zone, More Than 50 Ways to Help You Find the Best Diet for You*. Running Press, Philadelphia, Pennsylvania.

Rona, R.J., Keil, T., Summers, C., Gislason, D. *et al.* (2007) 'The prevalence of food allergy: a meta-analysis.' *Journal of Allergy and Clinical Immunology*, **120**(3): 638–646.

Rossignol, D.A. and Bradstreet, J. (2008) 'Evidence of mitochondrial dysfunction in autism and implications for treatment.' *American Journal of Biochemistry and Biotechnology*, **4**(2): 208–217.

Rowe, K.S. (1988) 'Synthetic food colourings and "hyperactivity": a double-blind crossover study.' *Australasian Paediatric Journal*, **24**(2): 143–147.

Russell. R. and Taegtmeyer, H. (1991) 'Pyruvate carboxylation prevents the decline in contractile function of rat hearts oxidizing acetoacetate.' *American Journal of Physiology*, **257**: E212–219.

Ryle, G. (1949) *The Concept of Mind*. Hutchinson: London.

Sackett, D.L., Haynes, R.B., Tugwell, P. and Guyatt, G.H. (1991) *Clinical Epidemiology: A Basic Science for Clinical Medicine*. Lippincott Williams & Wilkins: Philadelphia.

Sampath, A., Kossoff, E.H., Furth, S.L., Pyzik, P.L. and Vining, E.P.G. (2007) 'Kidney stones and the ketogenic diet: risk factors and prevention.' *Journal of Child Neurology*, **22**(4): 375–378.

Sandhu, M., White, I. and McPherson, K. (2001) 'Systematic review of the prospective cohort studies on meat consumption and colorectal cancer risk: a meta-analytical approach.' *Cancer Epidemiology, Biomarkers and Prevention*, **10**: 439–446.

Sankar, R. and Sotero de Menezes, M. (1999) 'Metabolic and endocrine aspects of the ketogenic diet.' *Epilepsy Research*, **37**: 191–201.

Savage, D.F. and Stroud, R.M. (2007) 'Structural basis of aquaporin inhibition by mercury.' *Journal of Molecular Biology*, **368**: 607–617.

Schaible, U.E. and Kaufmann, S.H.E. (2007) 'Malnutrition and infection: complex mechanisms and global impacts.' *PLOS Medicine*, **4**(5): e115, doi:10.1371/journal.pmed.0040115.t001.

Schenk, S. and Horowitz, J.F. (2007) 'Acute exercise increases triglyceride synthesis in skeletal muscle and prevents fatty acid-induced insulin resistance.' *The Journal of Clinical Investigation*, **117**(6): 1690–1697.

Schmidt, M.A. (1997) *Smart Fats: How Dietary Fats and Oils Affect Mental, Physical and Emotional Intelligence*. North Atlantic Publishing: Berkeley, California.

Schoenthaler, S.J. and Bier, I.D. (2000) 'The effect of vitamin-mineral supplementation on juvenile delinquency among American schoolchildren: a randomized, double-blind placebo-controlled trial.' *Journal of Alternative and Complementary Medicine*, **6**(1): 7–17.

Schonwald, A. (2008) 'ADHD and food additives revisited.' *AAP Grand Rounds*, **19**: 17.

Schweizer, U., Brauer, A.U., Kohrle, J., Nitsch, R. and Savaskan, N.E. (2004) 'Selenium and brain function: a poorly recognized liaison.' *Brain Research Reviews*, **45**: 164–178.

Segurado, R., Conroy, J., Meally, E., Fitzgerald, M., Gill, M. and Gallagher, L. (2005) 'Confirmation of association between autism and the mitochondrial aspartate/glutamate carrier SLC25A12 gene on chromosome 2q31.' *American Journal of Psychiatry*, **162**(11): 2182–2184.

Seroussi, K. (1999) *Unraveling the Mystery of Autism and Pervasive Developmental Disorder: A Mother's Story of Research and Recovery*. Broadway Books: New York.

Seroussi, K. and Lewis, L.S. (2008) *The Encyclopaedia of Dietary Interventions for the Treatment of Autism and Related Disorders*. Available to order at www.autismndi.com.

Sever, Y., Ashkenazi, A., Tyano, S. and Weizman, A. (1997) 'Iron treatment in children with ADHD: a preliminary report.' *Neuropsychobiology*, **35**: 178–180.

Shamaly, H., Hartman, C., Pollack, S., Hujerat, M. *et al.* (2007) 'Tissue transglutaminase antibodies are a useful serological marker for the diagnosis of celiac disease in patients with Down syndrome.' *Journal of Pediatric Gastroenterology and Nutrition*, **44**(5): 583–586.

Shannon, M. and Graef, J.W. (1997) 'Lead intoxication in children with pervasive developmental disorders.' *Journal of Toxicology and Clinical Toxicology*, **34**: 177–182.

Shapiro, R. (2008) *Suckers: How Alternative Medicine Makes Fools of Us All*. Harvill Secker, Random House: London.

Shattock, P., Carr, K. and Whiteley, P. (2007) 'Progress in understanding the role for organophosphate insecticides in the causation of autism and related spectrum disorders.' *The Autism File*, Winter: 40–45.

Shaw, W. (2008) 'Porphyrin testing and heavy metal toxicity: unresolved questions and concerns.' Unpublished document, available from: www.greatplainslaboratory.com.

Shoffner, J., Hyams, L.C. and Langley, G.N. (2008) 'Oxidative phosphorylation (OXPHOS) defects in children with autistic spectrum disorders.' Paper [IN1-1.004], American Academy of Neurology Meeting, Integrated Neuroscience Session, 13 April. Available from: www.abstracts2view.com/aan2008chicago/view.php?nu=AAN08L_IN1-1.004.

Shore, S. and Rastelli, L.G. (2006) *Understanding Autism for Dummies*. John Wiley & Sons: Chichester

Shulman, K.I. and Walker, S.E. (1999) 'Refining the MAOI diet: tyramine content of pizzas and soy products.' *Journal of Clinical Psychiatry*, **60**: 191–193.

Sicherer, S.H. (2002) 'Clinical update on peanut allergy.' *Annals of Allergy Asthma and Immunology*, **88**(4): 350–361.

Sicile-Kira, C. (2006) *Autism Spectrum Disorders: The Complete Guide to Understanding Autism, Asperger's Syndrome, Pervasive Developmental Disorder, and Other ASDs*. Perigree Books: New York.

Sidhu, H., Allison, M.J., Chow, J.-M., Clark, A. and Peck, A.B. (2001) 'Rapid reversal of hyperoxaluria in a rat model following probiotic administration of Oxalobacter formigenes.' *Journal of Urology*, **166**: 1487–1491.

Sidhu, H.B., Hoppe, H., Albrecht, K., Tenbrock, S. *et al.* (1998) 'Absence of *Oxalobacter formigenes* in cystic fibrosis patients: a risk factor for hyperoxaluria.' *Lancet*, **352**: 1026–1029.

Simopoulos, A.P. and Salem, N. Jr (1989) 'N-3 fatty acids in eggs from range-fed greek chickens.' Letter to the editor, *New England Journal of Medicine*, **321**: 1412.

Sinn, N. (2007) 'Physical fatty acid deficiency signs in children with ADHD symptoms.' *Prostaglandins, Leukotrienes and Essential Fatty Acids*, **77**: 109–115.

Smith, Q.R. (2000) 'Transport of glutamate and other amino acids at the blood-brain barrier.' *Journal of Nutrition*, **130**: 1016S–1022S.

Smith, W.E. (1975) *Minamata: The Story of the Poisoning of a City, and the People Who Choose to Carry the Burden of Courage*. Holt, Rinehart and Winston: New York.

Smith, W.B., Thompson, D., Kummerow, M., Quinn, P. and Gold, M.S. (2004) 'A2 milk is allergenic' (letter). *Medical Journal of Australia*, **181**(10): 574.

Sobanski, E., Marcus, A., Hennighausen, K., Hebebrand, J. and Schmidt, M.H. (1999) 'Further evidence for a low body weight in male children and adolescents with Asperger's disorder.' *European Child and Adolescent Psychiatry*, **8**(4): 312–314.

Sogut, S., Zoroglu, S.S., Ozyurt, H., Yilmaz, H.R. *et al.* (2003) 'Changes in nitric oxide levels and antioxidant enzyme activities may have a role in the pathophysiological mechanisms involved in autism.' *Clinica Chimica Acta*, **331**(1–2): 111–117.

Soloff, L. (1970) 'Arrhythmias following infusions of fatty acids.' *American Heart Journal*, **80**: 671–675.

Spaenij-Dekking, L., Kooy-Winkelaar, Y. and Koning, F. (2005) 'The Ethiopian cereal tef in celiac disease.' *New England Journal of Medicine*, **353**(16): 1748–1749.

Spencer, J.W. and Jacobs, J.J. (eds) (2003) *Complementary and Alternative Medicine: An Evidence-Based Approach*. Mosby Inc.: St.Louis, Missouri.

Speth, J.D. and Spielmann, K.A. (1983) 'Energy source, protein metabolism, and hunter-gatherer subsistence strategies.' *Journal of Anthropological Archaeology*, **2**: 1–31.

Starobrat-Hermelin, B. and Kozielec, T. (1997) 'The effects of magnesium physiological supplementation on hyperactivity in children with ADHD: positive response to magnesium oral loading test.' *Magnesium Research*, **10**: 149–156.

Stefansson, V. (1944) *Arctic Manual*. MacMillan Publishing: New York.

Stefansson, V. (1949) *Not by Bread Alone*. MacMillan Publishing: New York.

Stephan, D.A. (2008) 'Unravelling autism' (Commentary). *American Journal of Human Genetics*, **82**: 7–9.

Sternberg, E.M. (2001) *The Balance Within: The Science Connecting Health and Emotions*. W.H. Freeman: New York.

Stone, T. and Darlington, G. (2000) *Pills, Potions, Poisons: How Drugs Work*. Oxford University Press: Oxford.

Suh, J.H., Walsh, W.J., McGinnis, W.R., Lewis, A. and Ames, B.N. (2008) 'Altered sulfur amino acid metabolism in immune cells of children diagnosed with autism.' *American Journal of Biochemistry and Biotechnology*, **4**(2): 105–113.

Sun, Z., Cade, R.J., Fregly, M.J. and Privette, R.M. (1999) 'ß-casomorphin induces fos-like immunoreactivity in discrete brain regions relevant to schizophrenia and autism.' *Autism*, **3**(1): 67–83.

Sundram, K., Karupaiah, T. and Hayes, K.C. (2007) 'Stearic acid-rich interesterified fat and trans-rich fat raise the LDL/HDL ratio and plasma glucose relative to palm olein in humans.' *Nutrition and Metabolism*, **4**: 3. doi:10.1186/1743-7075-4-3.

Swallow, D.M. (2003) 'Genetic influences on carbohydrate digestion.' *Nutrition Research Reviews*, **16**: 37–43.

Swift, I., Paquette, D., Davison, K. and Saeed, H. (1999) 'Pica and trace element deficiencies in adults with developmental disabilities.' *The British Journal of Developmental Disabilities*, **45**(2), 111–117.

Swinburn, B. (2004) 'Beta casein A1 and A2 in milk and human health.' *Report to New Zealand Food Safety Authority*. Available from: www.salmon.org.nz.

Sykes, N.H. and Lamb, J.A. (2007) 'Autism: the quest for the genes.' *Expert Reviews in Molecular Medicine*, **9**(24): 1–15.

Szpir, M. (2006) 'Tracing the origins of autism: a spectrum of new studies.' *Environmental Health Perspectives*, **114**(7): A412–A418.

Tallian, K.B., Nahita, M.C. and Tsao, C.Y. (1998) 'Role of the ketogenic diet in children with intractable seizures.' *Annals of Pharmacotherapy*, **32**(3): 349–361.

Tani, P., Lindberg, N., Nieminen-von Wendt, T., von Wendt, L. *et al.* (2003) 'Insomnia is a frequent finding in adults with Asperger syndrome.' *BMC Psychiatry*, **3**: 12, available from www.biomedcentral.com/1471-244X/3/12.

Taubes, G. (2007) *The Diet Delusion*. Vermillion Press: London.

Taylor, E.N., Stampfer, M.J. and Curhan, G.C. (2005) 'Obesity, weight gain, and the risk of kidney stones.' *JAMA*, **293**: 455–462.

Thomson, C.D. and Robinson, M.F. (1980) 'Selenium in human health and disease with emphasis on those aspects peculiar to New Zealand.' *American Journal of Clinical Nutrition*, **33**: 303–323.

Tickner, J.A., Schettler, T., Guidotti, T., McCally, M. and Rossi, M. (2001) 'Health risks posed by use of Di-2-ethylhexyl phthalates (DEHP) in PVC medical devices: a critical review.' *American Journal of Industrial Medicine*, **39**(1): 100–111.

Tierney, E., Nwokoro, N.A. and Kelley, R.I. (2000) 'Behavioral phenotype of RSH/Smith-Lemli-Opitz syndrome.' *Mental Retardation and Developmental Disabilities Research Reviews*, **6**: 131–134.

Tierney, E., Nwokoro, N.A., Porter, F.D., Freund, L.S., Ghuman, J.K. and Kelley, R.I. (2001) 'Behavior phenotype in the RSH/Smith-Lemli-Opitz syndrome.' *American Journal of Medical Genetics*, **98**: 191–200.

Tierney, E., Bukelis, I., Thompson, R.E., Ahmed, K. *et al.* (2006) 'Abnormalities of cholesterol metabolism in autism spectrum disorders.' *American Journal of Medical Genetics B: Neuropsychiatric Genetics,* **141**: 666–668.

Tordjman, S., Anderson, G.M., Pichard, N., Charbuy, H. and Touitou, Y. (2005) 'Nocturnal excretion of 6-sulphatoxymelatonin in children and adolescents with autistic disorder.' *Biological Psychiatry,* **57**(1): 134–138.

Torres, R.J. and Puig, J.G. (2007) 'Hypoxanthine-guanine phosophoribosyltransferase (HPRT) deficiency: Lesch-Nyhan syndrome.' *Orphanet Journal of Rare Diseases,* **2**: 48. doi:10.1186/1750-1172-2-48.

Torsdottir, G., Hreidarsson, S., Kristinsson, J., Snaedal, J. and Johannesson, T. (2005) 'Ceruloplasmin, superoxide dismutase and copper in autistic patients.' *Basic & Clinical Pharmacology & Toxicology,* **96**: 146–148.

Trevarthen, C. and Aitken, K.J. (2001) 'Infant intersubjectivity: research, theory, and clinical applications.' *Journal of Child Psychology and Psychiatry,* **42**(1): 3–48.

Triumph Dining (2007) *The Essential Gluten-Free Grocery Guide.* Arlington, Virginia. Available from: www.triumphdining.com/index.aspx.

Triumph Dining (2008) *The Essential Gluten-Free Restaurant Guide* (3rd edn). Arlington, Virginia. Available from: www.triumphdining.com/index.aspx.

Trushina, E. and McMurray, C.T. (2007) 'Oxidative stress and mitochondrial dysfunction in neurodegenerative diseases.' *Neuroscience,* **145**: 1233–1248.

Tsai, L. (2001) *Taking the Mystery Out of Medications in Autism/Asperger's Syndromes.* Future Horizons: Arlington, Texas.

Tsumura, Y., Ishimitsu, S., Kaihara, A., Yoshii, K., Nakamura, Y. and Tonoga, Y. (2001) 'Di(2-ethylhexyl) phthalates contamination of retail packed lunches caused by PVC gloves used in the preparation of foods.' *Food Additives and Contaminants,* **18**(6): 569–579.

Tsumura, Y., Hirota, N., Tokura, H., Sone, Y. *et al.* (2005) 'Comparison of carbohydrate digestion between Japanese and Polish healthy subjects.' *Journal of Physiological Anthropology and Applied Human Science,* **24**(4): 507–509.

Turner, P.C., Rothwell, J.A., White, K.L.M., Gong, Y.-Y., Cade, J.E. and Wild, C.P. (2008) 'Urinary deoxynivalenol is correlated with cereal intake in individuals from the United Kingdom.' *Environmental Health Perspectives,* **116**(1): 21–25.

Uyanik, O., Dogangun, B., Kayaalp, L., Korkmaz, B. and Dervent, A. (2006) 'Food faddism causing vision loss in an autistic child.' *Child: Care, Health and Development,* **32**(5): 601–602.

Vader, L.W., de Ru, A., van der Wal, Y., Kooy, Y.M. *et al.* (2002) 'Specificity of tissue transglutaminase explains cereal toxicity in celiac disease.' *Journal of Experimental Medicine,* **195**(5): 643–649.

Vader, L.W., Stepniak, D.T., Bunnik, E.M., Kooy, Y.M. *et al.* (2003) 'Characterization of cereal toxicity for celiac disease patients based on protein homology in grains.' *Gastroenterology,* **125**(4): 1105–1113.

Valicenti-McDermott, M., McVicar, K., Rapin, I., Wershil, B.K., Cohen, H. and Shinnar, S. (2006) 'Frequency of gastrointestinal symptoms in children with autistic spectrum disorders and association with family history of autoimmune disease.' *Journal of Developmental and Behavioral Pediatrics,* **27**: 128–136.

Vanli, L., Yilmaz, E., Tokatli, A. and Anlar, B. (2006) 'Phenylketonuria in pediatric neurology practice: a series of 146 cases.' *Journal of Child Neurology,* **21**: 987–990.

Varner, J.A., Jensen, K.F., Horvath, W. and Isaacson, R.L. (1998) 'Chronic administration of aluminum-fluoride or sodium-fluoride to rats in drinking water: alterations in neuronal and cerebrovascular integrity.' *Brain Research,* **784**(1–2): 284–298.

Vazirian, S., Abolfazli, R., Mirbagheri, A., Hosseini, M.E. and Zabihi, A. (2007) 'Relationship between autism and celiac disease: a case-control study.' *American Academy of Neurology Annual Conference Presentation,* May 2007.

Verkman, A.S., Binder, D.K., Bloch, O., Auguste, K. and Papadopoulos, M.C. (2006) 'Three distinct roles of aquaporin-4 in brain function revealed by knockout mice.' *Biochimica et Biophysica Acta,* **1758**: 1085–1093.

Verrotti, A., Greco, R., Morgese, G. and Chiarelli, F. (1999) 'Carnitine deficiency and hyperammonemia in children receiving valproic acid with and without other anticonvulsant drugs.' *International Journal of Clinical and Laboratory Research*, **29**(1): 36–40.

Vethaak, A.D., Lahr, J., Schrap, S.M., Belfroid, A.C. *et al.* (2005) 'An integrated assessment of estrogenic contamination and biological effects in the aquatic environment of The Netherlands.' *Chemosphere*, **59**(4): 511–524.

Vilaseca, M.A., Briones, P., Ferrer, I., Campistol, J. *et al.* (1993) 'Controlled diet in phenylketonuria may cause serum carnitine deficiency.' *Journal of Inherited Metabolic Disease*, **16**(1): 101–104.

Walker, S.E., Shulman, K.I., Tailor, S.A. and Gardner, D. (1996) 'Tyramine content of previously restricted foods in monoamine oxidase inhibitor diets.' *Journal of Clinical Psychopharmacology*, **16**: 383–388.

Walker, S.J., Segal, J. and Aschner, M. (2006) 'Cultured lymphocytes from autistic children and non-autistic siblings up-regulate heat shock protein RNA in response to thimerosal challenge.' *Neurotoxicology*, **27**(5): 685–692.

Wallace, D.C. (2005) 'The mitochondrial genome in human adaptive radiation and disease: on the road to therapeutics and performance enhancement.' *Gene*, **354**: 169–180.

Wallace, T.M. and Matthews, D.R. (2004) 'recent advances in the monitoring and management of diabetic ketoacidosis.' *Clinical Laboratory Science*, **18**: 139–145.

Walsh, W.J., Isaacson, H.R., Rehman, F. and Hall, A. (1997) 'Elevated blood copper/zinc ratios in assaultive young males.' *Physiology & Behavior*, **62**(2): 327–329.

Waring, R.H. and Klovrza, L.V. (2000) 'Sulphur metabolism in autism.' *Journal of Nutritional and Environmental Medicine*, **10**(1): 25–32.

Warskulat, U., Flogel, U., Jacoby, C., Hartwig, H.-G. *et al.* (2004) 'Taurine transporter knockout depletes muscle taurine levels and results in severe skeletal muscle impairment but leaves cardiac function uncompromised.' *The FASEB Journal*, **18**(3): 577–579.

Whiteley, P., Rodgers, J., Savery, D. and Shattock, P. (1999) 'A gluten-free diet as an intervention for autism and associated spectrum disorders: preliminary findings.' *Autism*, **3**: 45–65.

Wiecha, J.L., Finkelstein, D., Troped, P.J., Fragala, M. and Peterson, K.E. (2006a) 'School vending machine use and fast-food restaurant use are associated with sugar-sweetened beverage intake in youth.' *Journal of the American Dietetic Association*, **106**(10): 1624–1630.

Wiecha, J.L., Peterson, K.E., Ludwig, D.S., Kim, J., Sobol, A. and Gortmaker, S.L. (2006b) 'When children eat what they watch: impact of television viewing on dietary intake in youth.' *Archives of Pediatrics and Adolescent Medicine*, **160**(4): 436–442.

Wier, M.L., Yoshida, C.K., Odouli, R., Grether, J.K. and Croen, L.A. (2006) 'Congenital anomalies associated with autism spectrum disorders.' *Developmental Medicine and Child Neurology*, **48**: 500–507.

Wilder, R.M. (1921) 'The effect of ketonemia on the course of epilepsy.' *Mayo Clinic Bulletin*, **2**: 307–308.

Wilens, T.E. (2008) *Straight Talk About Psychiatric Medication for Kids* (3rd edn). Guildford Press: New York.

Will, E.J. and Bijvoet, O.L.M. (1979) 'Primary oxalosis: clinical and biochemical response to high-dose pyridoxine therapy.' *Metabolism*, **28**: 542–548.

Williams, A.W. and Wilson, D.M. (1990) 'Dietary intake, absorption, metabolism, and excretion of oxalate.' *Seminars in Nephrology*, **10**(1): 2–8.

Williams, H.E. and Smith, L.H. (1968) 'Disorders of oxalate metabolism.' *American Journal of Medicine*, **45**: 715–735.

Williams, M.S. (2003) 'Can genomic deliver on the promise of improved results and reduced costs?: background and recommendations for health insurers.' *Disease Management and Health Outcomes*, **11**(5): 277–290.

Williams, R.J. (1998) *Biochemical Individuality: Basis for the Genetotrophic Concept* (2nd edn). Keats Publishing: Wilton, Connecticut.

Wing, R.R., Vazquez, J. and Ryan, C. (1995) 'Cognitive effects of ketogenic weight reducing diets.' *International Journal of Obesity Related Metabolic Disorders*, **19**: 811–816.

Wintour, E.M. and Henry, B.A. (2006) 'Glycerol transport: an additional target for obesity therapy?' *TRENDS in Endocrinology and Metabolism*, **17**(3): 77–78.

Wolcott, W.L. and Fahey, T. (2002) *The Metabolic Typing Diet* (2nd edn). Broadway Books: New York.

Wright, B., Brzozowski, A.M., Calvert, E., Farnworth, H. *et al.* (2005) 'Is the presence of urinary indolyl-3-acryloylglycine associated with autism spectrum disorder?' *Developmental Medicine and Child Neurology*, **47**: 190–192.

WWF (World Wildlife Fund) (2003) *Contamination: The Results of WWF's Biomonitoring Survey.* Available from: www.wwf.org.uk/filelibrary/pdf/biomonitoringresults.pdf.

WWF (World Wildlife Fund) (2007) *Chain of Contamination: The Food Link (Fact Sheet): Alkylphenols (Octylphenols and Nonylphenol Isomers).* Available from: www.wwf.org.uk/filelibrary/contamination.pdf

Xia, Y., Hill, K.E., Byrne, D.W., Xu, J. and Burk, R.F. (2005) 'Effectiveness of selenium supplements in a low-selenium area of China.' *American Journal of Clinical Nutrition*, **81**: 829–834.

Yamamoto, T., Kuramoto, H. and Kadowaki, M. (2007) 'Downregulation in aquaporin 4 and aquaporin 8 expression of the colon associated with the induction of allergic diarrhea in a mouse model of food allergy.' *Life Sciences*, **81**: 115–120.

Yang, Y., He, M., Cui, H., Bian, L. and Wang, Z. (2000) 'The prevalence of lactase deficiency and lactose intolerance in Chinese children of different ages.' *Chinese Medical Journal* (English), **113**(12): 1129–1132.

Young, G. and Conquer, J. (2005) 'Omega-3 fatty acids and neuropsychiatric disorders.' *Reproduction Nutrition Development*, **45**: 1–28.

Young, R.J. and Huffman, S. (2003) 'Probiotic use in children.' *Journal of Pediatric Health Care*, **17**: 277–283.

Yoshimura, I., Sasaki, A., Akimoto, H. and Yoshimura, N. (1989) '[A case of congenital myotonic dystrophy with infantile autism].' *No To Hattatsu*, **21**(4): 379–384.

Yu, H. and Patel, S.B. (2005) 'Recent insights into the Smith-Lemli-Opitz syndrome.' *Clinical Genetics*, **68**(5): 383–391.

Yussman, S.M., Ryan, S.A., Auinger, P. and Weitzman, M. (2004) 'Visits to complementary and alternative medicine providers by children and adolescents in the United States.' *Ambulatory Pediatrics*, **4**(5): 429–435.

Zafeiriou, D.I., Ververi, A., Salomons, G.S., Vargiami, E. *et al.* (2007) 'L-2-hydroxyglutaric aciduria presenting with severe autistic features.' *Brain and Development*, doi:10.1016/j.braindev.2007.09.005.

Zhou, J., Kong, H., Hua, X., Xiao, M., Ding, J. and Hu, G. (2008) 'Altered blood-brain barrier integrity in adult aquaporin-4 knockout mice.' *NeuroReport*, **19**: 1–5.

Subject Index

Author Index